THIRD EDITION

Pharmacy Technician Certification

Review *and* Practice Exam

Barbara Lacher

AMERICAN SOCIETY OF HEALTH-SYSTEM PHARMACISTS®

Any correspondence regarding this publication should be sent to the publisher, American Society of Health-System Pharmacists, 7272 Wisconsin Avenue, Bethesda, MD 20814, attn: Special Publishing. Produced in conjunction with the ASHP Publications Production Center.

The information presented herein reflects the opinions of the contributors and reviewers. It should not be interpreted as an official policy of ASHP or as an endorsement of any product.

This review book is not sponsored or endorsed by the Pharmacy Technician Certification Board (PTCB). Although every effort has been made on behalf of the authors, editor, and publisher to provide an extensive review, comprehension of the material included in this text and the practice exam does not guarantee successful completion of the PTCB national certification examination or any other examination. The practice exam represents the opinions of the authors and editors of this work and has not been field-tested or reviewed by PTCB.

The authors, editor, and publisher of this work have made a conscientious effort to provide the reader with accurate and up-to-date information, but the nature of the information is evolving, and may be subject to change due to the dynamic nature of drug information and drug distribution systems. This information should be used solely in preparation for the certification exam or other academic purposes. No information contained in this text should be used to provide patient care.

Director, Special Publishing: Jack Bruggeman

Acquisitions Editor: Rebecca Olson

Senior Editorial Project Manager: Dana Battaglia

Production Editor: Publication Services

Design: Publication Services

ISBN 978-1-58528-208-1

Library of Congress Cataloging-in-Publication Data

Lacher, Barbara E.
Pharmacy technician certification review and practice exam / Barbara Lacher. — 3rd ed.
p. ; cm.
Rev. ed. of: Pharmacy technician certification review and practice exam / Linda Y. Fred. 2nd ed. c2005.
Companion v. to: Manual for pharmacy technicians. 4th ed. c2011.
Includes index.
ISBN 978-1-58528-208-1
1. Pharmacy technicians—Outlines, syllabi, etc. 2. Pharmacy technicians—Examinations, questions, etc. I. Fred, Linda. Pharmacy technician certification review and practice exam. II. American Society of Health-System Pharmacists. III. Manual for pharmacy technicians. IV. Title.
[DNLM: 1. Pharmacy—Programmed Instruction. 2. Pharmaceutical Services—Programmed Instruction. 3. Pharmacists' Aides—Programmed Instruction. QV 18.2]
RS122.95.P436 2011
615'.1076—dc22

2010041276

Contents

Preface

Pharmacy Technician Certification Review and Practice Exam, third edition, is a self-study guide that is designed to be a companion book to the *Manual for Pharmacy Technicians*, fourth edition. This book was designed to assist pharmacy technicians and pharmacy technician students who are preparing to take the Pharmacy Technician Certification Examination offered through the Pharmacy Technician Certification Board (PTCB) or other pharmacy technician examinations.

The first three sections of the book correspond with the three sections of the PTCB examination and utilize the knowledge statements of those sections as a basis for the learning objectives of the chapters. Chapters reviewing calculations and commonly prescribed medications have been updated, including new assessment questions. The conclusion of the book contains a Practice Exam. The number of self-assessment questions at the end of each chapter has doubled in this edition and the Practice Exam contains new questions as well.

The *TechPrep*™ CD program is packaged along with the book. The PTCB exam and other pharmacy technician certification exams are taken on computers at authorized testing centers. TechPrep™ helps readers prepare for the test experience with more than 1000 practice questions. Readers can create customized practice session functions or run through simulated exams. TechPrep also provides instant feedback and scoring so that users can immediately see where they need more practice. To get started, simply load the CD into your computer, and the menu will automatically appear.

As with all editions of this review manual, it is not intended to be used as a sole preparation guide for the certification exam. This book should be used in conjunction with the *Manual for Pharmacy Technicians*, fourth edition, and other study materials recommended by the PTCB.

Barbara Lacher
2010

For additional resources and information, please visit www.ashp.org/techreview.

Contributors

ASHP gratefully acknowledges the following individuals for their contribution to the *Manual for Pharmacy Technicians*, fourth edition, which served as the foundation for this publication.

Bonnie S. Bachenheimer, PharmD
Clinical Pharmacist, Drug Information
Advocate Lutheran General Hospital
Park Ridge, Illinois

Karen E. Bertch, PharmD, FCCP
Director, Formulary Development
Medication Management Group
Premier, Inc.
Lisle, Illinois

Susan P. Bruce, PharmD, BCPS
Associate Professor and Chair
Pharmacy Practice
Colleges of Medicine and Pharmacy
Northeastern Ohio Universities
Rootstown, Ohio

Margaret Byun, PharmD, MS
Assistant Director, Finance and Administration
Ambulatory Care Pharmacy Department
Clinical Assistant Professor of Pharmacy Practice
University of Illinois at Chicago College of Pharmacy
Chicago, Illinois

Diane L. Darvey, PharmD, JD
Alexandria, Virginia

Thomas C. Dowling, PharmD, PhD, FCP
Associate Professor
Vice Chair, Department of Pharmacy Practice and Science
University of Maryland School of Pharmacy
Baltimore, Maryland

Sandra F. Durley, RPh, PharmD
Associate Director, Ambulatory Care Pharmacy Department
Clinical Assistant Professor
University of Illinois at Chicago College of Pharmacy
Chicago, Illinois

John F. Falkenholm, PharmD
Pharmacy Manager
Advocate Lutheran General Hospital
Park Ridge, Illinois

Alice J. A. Gardner, BSc, PhD
Associate Professor of Pharmacology
School of Pharmacy–Worcester
Massachusetts College of Pharmacy and Health Sciences
Worcester, Massachusetts

David R. Karls, RPh, MBA
Community Pharmacist
Fuquay Varina, North Carolina

Jacqueline Z. Kessler, MS, FASHP
Clinical Pharmacist
Advocate Lutheran General Hospital
Park Ridge, Illinois

Thomas E. Kirschling, PharmD, MS
Manager, Pharmacy Operations
University of Pittsburg Medical Center Presbyterian
Pittsburgh, Pennsylvania

Jane E. Krause, BS Pharm, MS, RPh
Clinical Associate Professor of Pharmacy Practice
Purdue University College of Pharmacy
West Lafayette, Indiana

Christopher M. Kutza, PharmD
Pharmacy Manager
Advocate Lutheran General Hospital
Park Ridge, Illinois

Steven Lundquist, PharmD
Clinical Director
Cardinal Health, Pharmacy Solutions
Marco Island, Florida

Scott M. Mark, PharmD, MS, MEd, MBA, MPH, FASHP, FACHE
Director of Pharmacy
Director, Pharmacy Practice Management Residency
University of Pittsburgh Medical Center
Associate Professor and Vice Chair of Pharmacy Systems
University of Pittsburgh School of Pharmacy
Pittsburgh, Pennsylvania

Mary B. McHugh, PharmD
Director, Pharmacy Technology
University of Montana College of Technology
Missoula, Montana

Jerrod Milton, Bsc Pharm, RPh
Vice President, Operations
Children's Hospital
Aurora, Colorado

Bertram A. Nicholas Jr., BS, MS, EdD, RPh
Assistant Dean for Experiential Education
Saint Joseph College School of Pharmacy
West Hartford, Connecticut

Michele F. Shepherd, PharmD, MS, BCPS, FASHP
Pharmacy Coordinator for Medical Education and Anticoagulation Services
Abbott Northwestern Hospital
Minneapolis, Minnesota

Miriam A. Mobley Smith, BS Pharm, PharmD
Interim Dean
Chicago State University College of Pharmacy
Chicago, Illinois

Daphne E. Smith-Marsh, PharmD, CDE
Clinical Assistant Professor/Clinical Pharmacist
University of Illinois at Chicago College of Pharmacy
Chicago, Illinois

Sheri Stensland, PharmD, AE-C, FAPhA
Associate Professor, Pharmacy Practice
Midwestern University–Chicago College of Pharmacy
Downers Grove, Illinois

JoAnn Stubbings, RPh, MHCA
Manager, Research and Public Policy
Clinical Associate Professor
Center for Pharmacoeconomic Research
University of Illinois at Chicago College of Pharmacy
Chicago, Illinois

Kara D. Weatherman, PharmD, BCNP, FAPhA
Clinical Assistant Professor of Pharmacy Practice
Purdue University College of Pharmacy
West Lafayette, Indiana

Chapter 1

Assisting the Pharmacist

Learning Outcomes

After completing this chapter, the technician should be able to:

- Define the terms *medication order* and *prescription,* and list the common means by which they are received by the pharmacy.
- Define commonly used pharmacy terms and abbreviations used in medication orders and prescriptions.
- List the required elements on a prescription or medication order.
- Define National Drug Code (NDC) numbers and put into proper order for transmittal.
- Verify correct Drug Enforcement Agency (DEA) numbers.
- Describe the steps required for proper prescription and medication order processing.
- Describe when a patient signature is required at the point of sale.
- Describe how prescriptions are transferred between pharmacies.
- Explain good compounding practices and aseptic technique.
- Give examples of drugs with Risk Evaluation and Mitigation Strategy (REMS).
- List and describe the equipment used in both sterile and nonsterile compounding.
- Describe the process utilized to prepare cytotoxic and hazardous drugs.
- Define laminar airflow workbenches (LAFW) and biological safety cabinets (BSC).

This chapter applies to Section I of the PTCB exam, Assisting the Pharmacist in Serving Patients.

- Describe the types of questions that may be answered by a pharmacy technician.
- List common references found in many pharmacies and what information might be found in each.

Medication Orders and Prescriptions Defined

Typically, the term *medication order* refers to a written request on a physician's order form or a transcribed verbal or telephone order in an inpatient setting. This order becomes part of the patient's medical record. The term *prescription* refers to a medication order on a prescription blank to be filled in an outpatient or ambulatory care setting. The two serve essentially the same purpose. They both represent a means of communication for the prescriber to give instruction to the dispenser of the medication or to those who will be administering the medication.

Pharmacy Terms and Abbreviations

Pharmacy personnel use a number of terms in their work. An understanding of these terms helps a technician to be efficient and capable.

Some of these terms define classifications of drugs. For example, technicians must be able to differentiate between *generic* and *brand name* drugs. A generic name describes a unique chemical entity and can be applied to that entity regardless of its manufacturer. A brand name is trademarked by a manufacturer to identify its particular "brand" of that chemical entity. For example, Ancef® is a brand name product of the generic entity cefazolin.

Another pair of terms used to categorize drugs is *legend* and *over-the-counter.* A legend drug, also called a prescription drug, is one that may not be dispensed to the public except on the order of a physician or other licensed prescriber. The term comes from the federal legend that appears on the packaging: "Federal law prohibits dispensing this medication without a prescription." Over-the-counter medications may be sold to the public without a prescription as long as they are properly labeled for home use.

One last term, *formulary,* is used in slightly different ways in institutional and retail settings. A formulary is a listing of approved drugs available for use. In a hospital, it refers to the drugs that are stocked by the pharmacy and approved for use in the facility. In the retail setting, the term is generally applied to an approved drug list associated with a particular benefit plan.

Pharmacy abbreviations are commonly used as a kind of shorthand in prescriptions and medication orders to convey information about directions for use. The abbreviations are then "translated" on the prescription label. Appendix A lists many commonly used pharmacy abbreviations.

The abbreviations for time and frequency of medication administration come from Latin phrases. Other commonly used abbreviations include those for routes of administration and those that designate units of measure. Lowercase Roman numerals are often used to denote a quantity, such as a number of tablets (i = one; ii = two). (See Chapter 14 of *Manual for Pharmacy Technicians* for a review of Roman numerals.)

Another subset of abbreviations is called *x-substitutions* and includes the well-known and widely recognized *Rx* symbol, meaning *prescription.* Other common x-substitutions are *dx* for *diagnosis* and *sx* for *symptoms.*

Abbreviations in medical records and in prescriptions are thought to be contributing factors in some medical errors. One important example is the use of the letter *U* to abbreviate units. Because a *U* might be misread as a zero if sloppily written—and could therefore result in a tenfold dosing error—the Institute for Safe Medication Practices recommends that it never be used as an abbreviation in prescriptions or medication orders; the word *units* should always be written out in its entirety. Other abbreviations that some consider unsafe are *q., qid,* and *qod,* which may be indistinguishable from each other if legibility is poor. These three abbreviations have been included in the chapter because they are still widely used.

Receiving and Processing Medication Orders in a Hospital

Medication orders come to the hospital pharmacy in various ways. They can be delivered to the pharmacy or one of its satellites in person or via some mechanical method, such as fax transmission or a pneumatic tube system. Orders may also be telephoned to the pharmacy by either the prescriber or an intermediary, such as a nurse. There are some legal restrictions on who may telephone in an order or a prescription, and who may receive that information in the pharmacy—particularly when controlled substances are involved.

Ideally, every medication order should contain the following elements:

- Patient name, hospital identification number, and room/bed location
- Generic drug name (using generic drug names is recommended, and many institutions have policies to this effect)
- Brand drug name (if a specific product is required)
- Route of administration (with some orders, the site of administration should also be included)
- Dosage form
- Dose/strength
- Frequency and duration of administration (if duration is pertinent—may be open-ended)
- Rate and time of administration, if applicable
- Indication for use of the medication
- Other instructions for the person administering the medication, such as whether it should be given with food or on an empty stomach
- Prescriber's name/signature and credentials (some hospitals require a printed name, physician number, or pager number in addition to the signature to assist with identification)
- Signature and credentials of person writing the order if other than prescriber
- Date and time of the order

When a new order is received, the first step is to ensure that the order is clear and complete. If information is missing—for example, the room number for the patient—the technician may be able to clarify the order without pharmacist intervention. Some clarifications, however, should involve the pharmacist. (See the discussion of which questions can be handled by a technician later in this chapter.)

Once orders are deemed clear and complete, they must be prioritized so that the most urgent orders are filled first. Prioritizing orders means comparing the urgency of new orders with the urgency of all the orders requiring attention. This ensures that those orders needed the most will be processed first. Technicians can prioritize orders by evaluating the route, time of administration, type of drug, intended use of the drug, and patient-specific circumstances.

A number of steps are involved in processing an order in the computer. First, the patient must be positively identified to avoid dispensing medication for the wrong patient; many institutions are now using bar code technology and electronic charting to facilitate accuracy. Second, the order is typically compared with the patient's existing medication profile, or a new profile is created for the patient. Then, the technician takes a number of order entry steps to update the patient's medication profile.

The following step-by-step process outlines a fairly typical medication order entry process. Systems vary somewhat, however, and this is simply an example of what the process flow might look like.

1. Enter the patient's name or medical record number and verify them to ensure that the correct patient record has been chosen.
2. Compare the order with the patient profile in detail to look for duplications, other possible problems, or to create the patient profile. Check for general appropriateness of the order; it should make sense in regard to patient profile information, such as the patient's age, allergies, and drugs currently being taken. The following information is appropriately found in the hospital pharmacy's patient profile, although system capabilities may limit access to some components:
   - Patient name and identification number
   - Date of birth, or age
   - Sex
   - Height and weight
   - Certain lab values, such as creatinine clearance
   - Admitting and secondary diagnoses (including pregnancy and lactation status)
   - Name of parent or guardian, if applicable
   - Room and bed number
   - Names of admitting and consulting physicians
   - Medication allergies; latex allergy; pertinent food allergies
   - Medication history (current and discontinued medications; medications from a previous admission in some instances)
   - Special considerations (eg, foreign language, disability)
   - Clinical comments (eg, therapeutic monitoring, counseling notes)
3. Enter the drug. Selecting the correct drug product requires a working knowledge of both brand names and generic names (although most computer systems can search for either name) and a sensible approach to interpreting orders when abbreviations are used. When in doubt about a drug name or an abbreviation, however, it is always better to clarify the order with the prescriber or the person who wrote the order. Patient safety must be protected, and it is dangerous to make assumptions when interpreting orders. Most pharmacies take special precautions to ensure accurate interpretation of prescriptions and medication orders involving look-alike and sound-alike drugs. With most pharmacy computer systems, drug products can be reviewed by scrolling through an alphabetical listing of the brand or generic names or by entering a code or mnemonic that is associated with the product name in the computer. Many computer systems alert the operator if he or she attempts to enter medications that interact with current orders, conflict with the patient's drug allergies, represent therapeutic duplications, or are nonformulary drugs. Many systems also check the dosage range and alert the pharmacist or technician if he or she enters a dose that exceeds the recommended dose for that patient. Although these alert systems help prevent errors, they are not always significant given the patient's unique situation. Therefore, the technician must consult the pharmacist when the alert is posted. Besides just choosing the "correct drug," as has been outlined in this section, some other related choices are included in this step. For example, if an intravenous (IV) medication is being entered, it might be necessary to choose the correct diluent into which the drug is to be mixed. Another decision involved in choosing the correct drug is the choice of the package type and size—bulk or unit dose, 15 gram tube or 30 gram tube, 100 ml bottle or 150 ml bottle.
4. Verify the dose to ensure that the correct amount has been entered.
5. Enter the administration schedule. In institutions, standard medication administration times are

generally set. These schedules are usually based on therapeutic issues or nursing efficiency or are designed to coordinate services, such as laboratory blood draws or therapy schedules. Standard administration schedules and protocols are usually agreed upon by pharmacy, nursing, and the hospital's medical staff. Many pharmacies have a written document, such as a policy, that staff can refer to when the appropriate administration time is unclear.

6. Enter any comments in the *clinical comments* field. The prescriber's directions for proper use of the medications must be conveyed clearly and accurately. Additional instructions for the caregiver are often entered into the pharmacy information system for presentation on one of the many documents printed from the profile (or for the nurses' use in an electronic system) or simply as additional information for the pharmacists' use at a later time. These special instructions might include storage information, such as the need to refrigerate, or special instructions, such as for chemotherapy drugs. Another example would be physician-specified parameters for use, such as, "hold if systolic BP less than 100 mm Hg," or "repeat in one hour if ineffective." These types of instructions would typically be displayed on the medication administration record (MAR) and also on the medication label.
7. Verify the prescriber name.
8. Fill and label the medication. Once the computer entry has been completed and labeling materials generated, the medication order must be filled with the correct quantity of the correct drug. During this step, the technician should carefully review the label against the order and the product to be used to make sure the correct product has been chosen. This is the final opportunity for the pharmacy to catch an error before dispensing to a patient care area. The medication order is then filled and left for the pharmacist to check. With few exceptions, this pharmacist check is legally required before dispensing any drug to a patient care area.

Receiving and Processing Prescriptions in an Outpatient Pharmacy

When welcoming a patient to the pharmacy, it is important to first identify him or her. If the patient has been to your pharmacy before, another piece of identifying information, such as date of birth, address, or phone number should be obtained to confirm the patient's identity. If the patient is bringing a prescription to you for the first time, he or she needs to be registered by obtaining the following information:

- Correct spelling of name
- Address and phone number(s)
- Insurance information from patient's insurance card
- Date of birth
- Any drug allergies
- Other prescriptions or over-the-counter (OTC) medications the patient takes regularly
- Significant health conditions

Prescriptions may be received directly from the patient or from the prescriber by telephone, fax, or electronic transmission.

Many pharmacies also accept refill requests over the Internet through a pharmacy Web page.

Obtaining payer information is an important step in receiving a prescription in the outpatient setting. This information is used for a number of purposes, including establishing the primary payer for the prescription, the patient's portion of the reimbursement (copay), and in some instances the drug formulary.

Reviewing a prescription for clarity and completeness is similar in the outpatient and the inpatient setting. The following prescription elements are typically present:

- Patient name
- Patient home address
- Date the prescription was written
- Drug name—either generic or brand
- Drug strength and dose to be administered
- Directions for use, including route of administration, frequency, and, as applicable, duration of use (some durations are open-ended)
- Quantity to be dispensed
- Number of refills to be allowed
- Substitution authority or refusal
- Signature and credentials of the prescriber, and DEA number, if required
- Reason for use, or indication (not generally required)

In an ambulatory practice, some special clarity and completeness issues must be considered. Receiving a prescription includes determining whether the prescription will be filled with generic or brand-name drugs. In many states when a prescriber uses "Dispense as Written" or DAW on a prescription blank, the brand name must be dispensed. The technician must know the requirements of their state.

> **? Pop Quiz!**
> If a prescription were ordered 1 tab qid, ac and hs, how would you write the label?

Assessing Order Authenticity

Screening prescriptions for potential forgeries, particularly those for controlled substances, is part of routine prescription processing. The technician should screen prescriptions for anything that looks unusual, such as a dispense quantity in excess of normal quantities or an unusual or unrecognizable signature. Any suspicious prescription should be discreetly presented to the pharmacist for further evaluation.

Prescription forgeries often take one of two forms: (1) erasure or overwriting of the strength or dispensing quantity of the drug (eg, changing a 3 to an 8), and (2) theft of preprinted prescription pads that may result in legitimate-looking prescriptions.

One thing a technician can do to help prevent prescription forgery is determine if a DEA number on a controlled substance prescription is valid. A valid DEA number consists of two letters and seven numbers, such as "BB 1 1 9 7 9 6 7." If the holder of the DEA number is a registrant, such as a physician or pharmacy, the first letter is an "A" or "B." If the holder of the DEA number is a mid-level practitioner, such as a qualified nurse practitioner, the first letter is an "M." The second letter is related to the registrant's name. In the case of a physician, it is the first letter of his or her last name.

The seven numbers are also used to determine a legitimate DEA number. The odd group—the 1st, 3rd, and 5th numbers in the sequence, and the even group—the 2nd, 4th, and 6th numbers—are added in the following manner so that the sum relates to the 7th number:

BB 1 1 9 7 9 6 **7**
Odd Group 1 + 9 + 9 = 19
Even Group 1 + 7 + 6 =14
Sum of odd (19) and 2 × even group (14 × 2)
= 19 + 28 = 47

The last digit of this odd/even group sum is the same as the last digit of the DEA number.

Prioritization of prescription processing in the outpatient pharmacy is generally an issue of customer service rather than patient care.

Prescription processing includes many of the same steps as medication order processing in the inpatient setting:

- Identifying the patient: It is important to make sure that prescriptions are filled for and dispensed to the correct patient. Proper attention needs to be paid to similar or identical names to make sure the medication is profiled on the right patient profile. Another important concern for the outpatient staff at this stage is to ensure that there is no forgery and that the individuals obtaining controlled substances are lawfully entitled to do so.
- Creating, maintaining, and reviewing patient profiles: A number of pieces of information are typically collected in the patient profile—some according to law (which varies from state to state) and some for efficiency and convenience purposes for both the pharmacy and the patient. These pieces of information include the following:
  - Patient's name and identification number
  - Age or date of birth
  - Home address and telephone number
  - Allergies
  - Principle diagnoses of patient
  - Primary health care providers for patient
  - Third-party payer(s) and other billing information
  - Over-the-counter medications and herbal supplements used by the patient
  - Prescription and refill history of the patient
  - Patient preferences (eg, child-resistant packaging waiver, preference for receiving prescriptions by mail)

Once the patient's profile is located or created and the existing information is verified, selecting the appropriate drug product is the next step in the order entry process. Most outpatient computer systems, like inpatient systems, allow drug product choice by typing in a mnemonic or by accessing an alphabetical listing of some sort. These are the typical prescription processing steps:

1. Enter the patient's medical record number or name and verify them. This safety step ensures that the drug is dispensed to the correct patient.

2. Enter or verify existing third-party billing information to ensure correct billing and copayment.
3. Compare the order with the patient profile in detail to identify duplications or other concerns.
4. Enter the prescription. A variety of information must be entered into the computer at this point, and systems vary as to the order in which it is entered. The following are required elements:
   - Physician's name
   - Directions for use, including special comments
   - Fill quantity
   - Initials of the pharmacist checking the prescription
   - Number of refills authorized

At the time of computer processing, an error message may interrupt transmission of the prescription to the third-party payer. The following are some common error messages and their meanings:

- *Refill Too Soon:* This message deals with refill prescriptions and the elapsed time between filling prescriptions. Typically, third parties allow patients to receive a 30-day supply of medications. If the patient attempts to refill a prescription within a significantly shorter period (eg, 15 days after the last prescription), the prescription cannot be processed without prior approval from the third-party payer.
- *Missing/Invalid Patient ID:* This or a similar message indicates that the patient who is entered into the pharmacy computer does not appear to be enrolled in the insurance program. On receiving this message, the technician should examine the patient information entered for mistakes. Perhaps the name was misspelled, identification number mistyped, or other required information left out. Because many insurance plans use a Pharmacy Benefit Manager (PBM) to manage their pharmacy services, the prescription may need to be processed under the name of the PBM instead of the name of the third-party payer.
- *Drug–Drug or Drug–Allergy Interaction:* Most pharmacy software will screen the patient profile for drug and allergy information. If interactions are detected, the program will alert the user. Some software will not only identify an interaction but also indicate its potential severity. A technician who receives a drug–drug or drug–allergy interaction message should alert the pharmacist to the problem.
- *Nonformulary/Not Covered:* Many third-party payers have formularies (lists of covered drugs). This message indicates that the drug is not covered, and payment will not be made for that drug. A technician who receives this message should alert the pharmacist.

5. Fill and label the prescription. The following components must generally appear on a prescription label, whether typed or computer-generated (may vary by state):
   - Patient's name
   - Date the prescription is being filled (or refilled)
   - Prescriber's name
   - Sequential prescription number
   - Name of the drug (including manufacturer if filled generically)
   - Quantity to be dispensed
   - Directions for use
   - Number of refills remaining (or associated refill period)

Labeling includes more than just the actual prescription label. The inpatient section of this chapter noted that labeling for inpatient use is often abbreviated or in a form of shorthand. For home use, however, this practice is not acceptable. Beyond the prescription label itself, auxiliary information is often included in the form of special labels affixed to the container or drug information leaflets for patients to read at home. Instructions for home use must include the following at a minimum:

- Administration directions (eg, "Take," "Insert," "Apply")
- Number of units constituting one dose and the dosage form (eg, 2 tablets)
- Route of administration (eg, "by mouth," "vaginally")
- How frequently or at what time (eg, "twice daily," "daily at 9 a.m.")
- Length of time to continue, if applicable (eg, "for 10 days," "until finished")
- Indication of purpose, if applicable (eg, "for pain," "for blood pressure")

At the time of dispensing, the pharmacist or technician must be sure the patient fully understands how to use the medication. This is also an appropriate time to consider language barriers, such as illiteracy or a primary language other than English.

NDC Numbers

NDC numbers are identification numbers used by drug manufacturers to identify their product. Each number is specific for a specific product. NDC numbers are used for verifying the correct drug has been used to fill the prescription and for remittance to third party companies.

- First group of numbers: represent the manufacturer. All products made by a specific manufacturer will have the same first number.
- Second group of numbers: represent the specific product.
- Third group of numbers: represent the package size.

In most cases, NDC numbers must be transmitted to a third party in a 5-4-2 configuration, even though the manufacturers do not always present them to us in that configuration. If we do not bill the NDC # correctly, the third party company's computer cannot read it correctly, and this could result in an error in payments, or no payment at all.

NDC Format	Corrected to 5-4-2 Format
0536-3922-01	**0**0536-3922-01
59930-1500-8	59930-1500-**0**8
38245-196-72	38245-**0**196-72

The NDC format is very specific, so placement of the zeros to create a 5-4-2 format is also very specific. *The zero is always placed at the beginning of the incorrect group of numbers.*

Pop Quiz!

What does the first letter of the DEA number signify?

Communication with Third Party Payers

Most claims for third party payers are handled by pharmacy benefits managers (see Chapter 3 of the Pharmacy Technician Certification Review) but if the pharmacy receives a message that the claim has been rejected, resolving these third party issues becomes a time-consuming part of the prescription process.

Collecting Payment and Patient Counseling

Technicians are usually involved in **point-of-sale** (POS) transactions, which involve checking out patients and collecting payment when prescription orders are complete.

1. Verify the patient's name and other identifying information to ensure the medication is being given to the correct patient.
2. Legal requirements regarding patient counseling must be met; offer to have the pharmacist visit with the patient if they would like counseling.
3. New patients must be given a copy of the pharmacy's patient privacy policy in compliance with Health Insurance Portability and Accountability Act (HIPAA) regulations.
4. The patients' signature is required when they receive the HIPAA information and by some states if they refuse counseling and by some third party payers when they take possession of the prescription.

Transferring Prescriptions

The laws regarding the transfer of prescriptions between pharmacies vary among states and among different classes of drugs. However, the pharmacist is always ultimately responsible for the information transferred. The transfer of a prescription to another pharmacy is usually initiated by a phone call from the pharmacy needing a transferred prescription. A technician may pull the original prescription from files or pull up the data on the computer, but the actual transfer of information is usually the responsibility of the pharmacist.

The same is true for prescriptions being transferred into the pharmacy. In this case, the process begins when a patient requests to transfer the prescription from another location. At that point, the technician must obtain from the patient as much information as possible about the prescription. At a minimum, the pharmacist needs the patient's name and the name of the pharmacy currently holding the prescription. If a patient brings in an old container, it may be useful to troubleshoot the label. For example, if the label indicates that there are no refills, the physician will have to be called to authorize the refill.

Handling Restricted Use Medications

There are certain medications that can only be prescribed and dispensed in a community or ambulatory care pharmacy under specific conditions due to special precautions regarding their use. The FDA requires a **Risk Evaluation and Mitigation Strategy (REMS)** when it determines that a strategy is necessary to ensure the benefits of using the drug outweigh the potential risks. Examples of drugs with REMS include: alosetron (Lotronex©), clozapine (Clozaril©, Fazaclo©), isotretinoin (Accutane©, Amnesteem©, Claravis©, Sotret©), thalidomide (Thalomid©), and dofetilide (Tikosyn©).

The FDA has designated other drugs that are required to be dispensed with **Medication Guides**. A Medication Guide is patient information approved by the FDA to help patients avoid serious adverse events, inform them about known serious side effects, and provide directions for use to promote adherence to the treatment. These are available for specific drugs or classes of drugs and must be dispensed with the prescription.[9] Common examples dispensed in community and ambulatory care pharmacies include nonsteroidal anti-inflammatory drugs (NSAID) and antidepressants.

Investigational Drugs

Investigational Drug services may be a form of services seen in a hospital or specialty pharmacy service. Before a study is approved to be conducted, a study protocol is developed, reviewed, and approved by the Institutional Review Board of the facility. In order to carry out a successful drug study there are specific requirements and procedures that must be followed. These include:

- proper storage
- record keeping
- inventory control
- preparation
- dispensing
- labeling of all investigational drugs

Good Compounding Practices

Chemicals for compounding are approved by the Food and Drug Administration (FDA); however, the practice of compounding is controlled by the individual state boards of pharmacy. Certain aspects of compounding and the role of the FDA were not clearly defined in federal law until, in 1997, the Food and Drug Administration Modernization Act (FDAMA) was passed. This legislation clearly defined the roles of both compounding pharmacies and the FDA. In the summer of 2002, however, the legislation was declared unconstitutional because of advertising restrictions. Nonetheless, the guidelines of the 1997 FDAMA still offer a structure for compounding pharmacists to follow until future legislation addresses the issue.

The *United States Pharmacopeia (USP 27)* offers guidelines for compounding. The following chapters of the *USP 27* review specific areas of compounding:

- Chapter 795 Pharmaceutical Compounding—Nonsterile Preparations
- Chapter 797 Pharmaceutical Compounding—Sterile Preparations
- Chapter 1075 Good Compounding Practices

The following are key areas of compounding:

1. Responsibility of the compounder
2. Compounding environment
3. Stability of compounded preparations
4. Ingredient selection
5. Compounded preparations
6. Compounding processes
7. Compounding records and documents
8. Material Safety Data Sheets (MSDS) file
9. Quality control
10. Patient counseling

? Pop Quiz!

NDC numbers are always transmitted in what format?

Responsibility of the Compounder

The compounder is responsible for all aspects of the compounding process, including, but not limited to, appropriately trained personnel and the key areas of Chapter 795 that follow. Special training is required for all personnel who prepare sterile products.

Compounding Environment

The compounding area should have adequate space for equipment and support materials. Controlled temperature and lighting are needed for chemicals and finished medications. The area must be kept clean for sanitary reasons and to prevent cross contamination. A sink with hot and cold running water is essential for handwashing and cleaning of equipment.

Stability of Compounded Preparations

Stability is defined in *USP-NF* as "the extent to which a preparation retains, within specified limits, and throughout its period of storage and use, the same properties and characteristics that are possessed at the time of compounding."

Primary packaging of the finished medication is of utmost importance. The choice of container is guided by the physical and chemical characteristics of the finished medication. Considerations such as light sensitivity and the medication binding to the container are examples of concern in maximizing stability.

Beyond-use labeling should be included on all medications (expiration dates apply to manufactured products). Examples of considerations for determining beyond-use dates include whether the medication is aqueous or nonaqueous, expiration date of the ingredients used, storage temperature, references documenting the stability of the finished medication, and the *USP*.

Ingredient Selection

Sources of ingredients vary widely. USP or National Formulary (NF) chemicals are the preferred source of chemicals for compounding. Other sources may be used, but the compounder has a responsibility to be certain the chemical meets purity and safety standards. Manufactured medications are another acceptable source of ingredients. It would be inappropriate to use any chemical withdrawn from use by the FDA.

Compounded Preparations

Preparations should contain at least 90%, but not more than 110%, of the labeled active ingredient, unless more restrictive laws apply. Compounding guidelines in *USP-NF* specifically address the following drug forms:

- Capsules, powders, lozenges, and tablets
- Emulsions, solutions, and suspensions
- Suppositories
- Creams, topical gels, ointments, and pastes

Compounding Processes

The goal of the compounding process is to "minimize error and maximize the prescriber's intent." The following list is a sample of areas to consider in the compounding process:

- Evaluation of the appropriateness of the prescription
- Calculations of the amount of ingredients
- Identification of equipment needed to properly compound the prescription
- Proper hand cleaning and gowning
- Evaluation of the final medication for weight variation, proper mixing, and consistency
- Proper notations in the compounding log
- Appropriate labeling of the final medication
- Properly clean and store all equipment

Compounding Records and Documents

USP Chapter 795 requires pharmacies to maintain a **formulation record** (also known as the **master formula**) and a **compounding record** for each compounded preparation. The goal of record-keeping is to allow another compounder to reproduce the same formulation at a later date. Two parts of the records and documentation are the *formula,* or *formulation record,* and the *batch log,* or *compounding record.*

The formulation record is a file of compounded preparations, much like a recipe. It would include chemicals in the formula, equipment needed to prepare the formula, and mixing instructions for preparing the formula.

The compounding record is the log (or record) of an actual batch being prepared. It would include manufacturers and lot numbers of chemicals used, the date of preparation, an internal identification number (commonly called lot number), a beyond-use date, and any other pertinent information regarding the preparation.

Quality Control

Quality control is a final check on the preparation to ensure safety and quality of the preparation. The compounder should evaluate the finished preparation both physically and by reviewing the compounding procedure to be certain the preparation is accurate. Discrepancies should be noted and evaluated to determine if the preparation is acceptable.

Patient Counseling

With any prescription, the patient should be counseled on the correct use of the medication. Compounded medications are often different in method of use or the type of dispensing container used, so special care should be taken to be certain the patient understands the proper use of the medication.

Equipment Used in Nonsterile Compounding

Compounding requires specialized equipment to obtain the best quality medications. An electronic balance is commonly used for speed and accuracy of measurement (see Figure 1-1). Graduates (ie, glass or plastic cylinders and conicals) are used to measure the volume of liquid ingredients (Figure 1-2). It is recommended to use the smallest graduate that will hold the volume to be measured. In addition, it is important to measure the volume of liquid accurately by placing the graduate on a stable surface (ie, counter top of work area) and read the measurement at the bottom of the meniscus.

An ointment slab (also called a "pill tile") is a square glass tile that is used for preparing and mixing creams and ointments. Similarly, many facilities use ointment paper (eg, pads of 12" × 12" disposable parchment paper) instead of an ointment slab because of convenience in reducing clean-up time (Figure 1-3).

Mortars and pestles are used to crush, grind, and blend various ingredients. The mortar is a deep bowl, and the pestle is a club-shaped tool that when stamped or pounded vertically into the well of the mortar causes the contents of the mortar to become pulverized (see Figure1-4). Mixing is usually achieved by moving the pestle in a circular motion in the mortar. Mortars are available in a variety of materials and sizes. Glass, porcelain, ceramic, and Wedgwood™ are commonly used. Wedgwood™ offers a rough surface to allow grinding and reduction of particle size but is very difficult to clean and thus prevent cross contamination of preparations. Glass and porcelain offer smooth, easily cleaned surfaces.

Ointment mills are commonly found in compounding pharmacies. Most have three rollers with small, adjustable spaces between the rollers (see Figure 1-5). When preparations pass through the rollers, particle size is reduced.

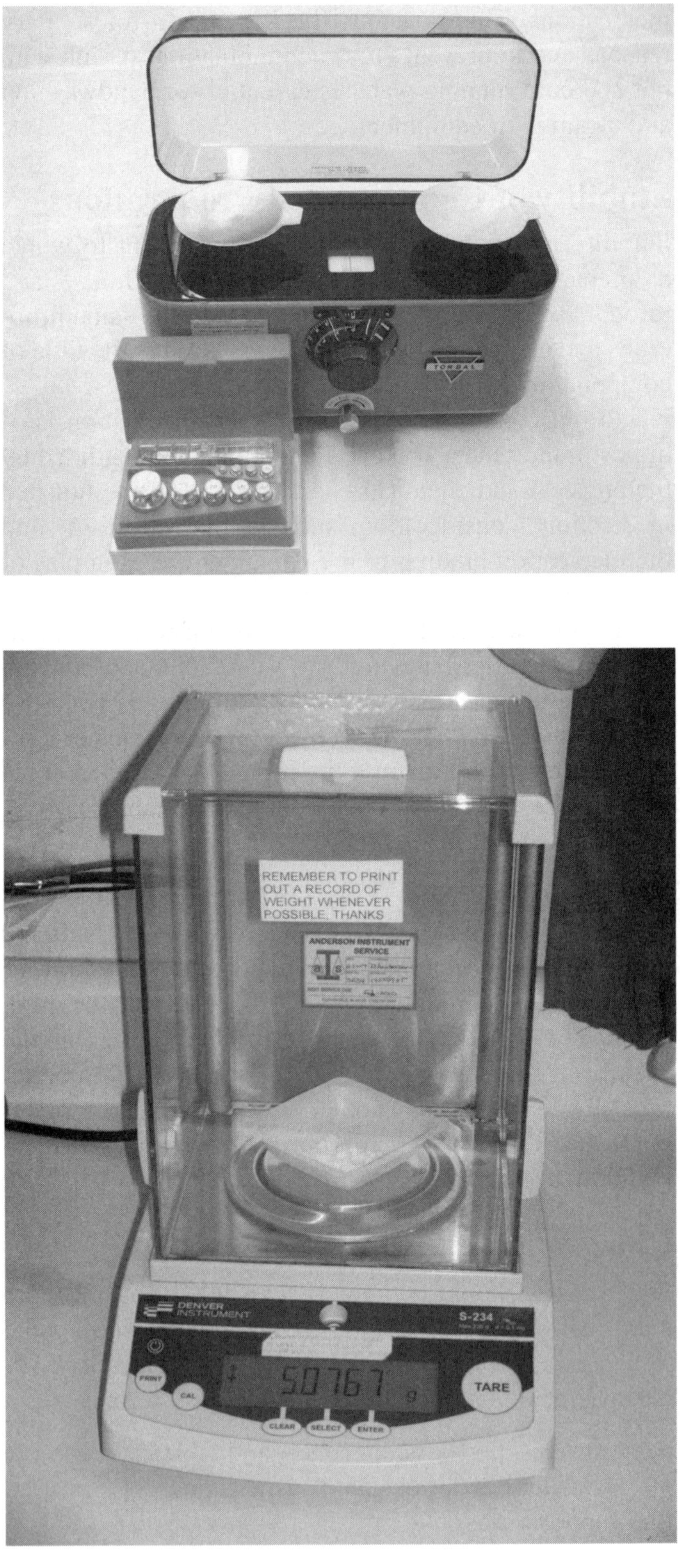

Figure 1-1. Electronic balance.

Parenteral Drug Administration

Medications can be administered to patients in numerous ways. Medications not given to patients by mouth (enterally) are referred to as *parenterally* administered. Parenteral administrations can include intravenous (IV), intramuscular (IM), and subcutaneous (SQ), or below the skin. IV solutions are commonly administered to patients as a means of replacing body fluids and as a vehicle for

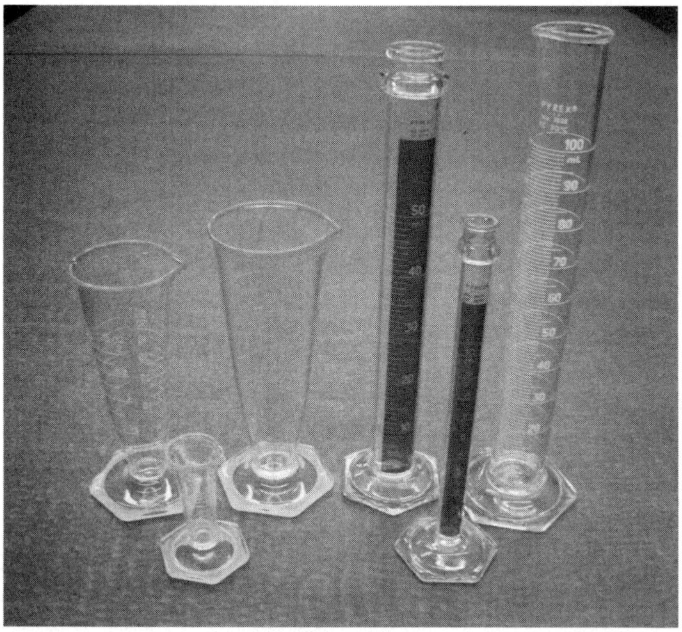

Figure 1–2. Graduated conicals and cylinders.

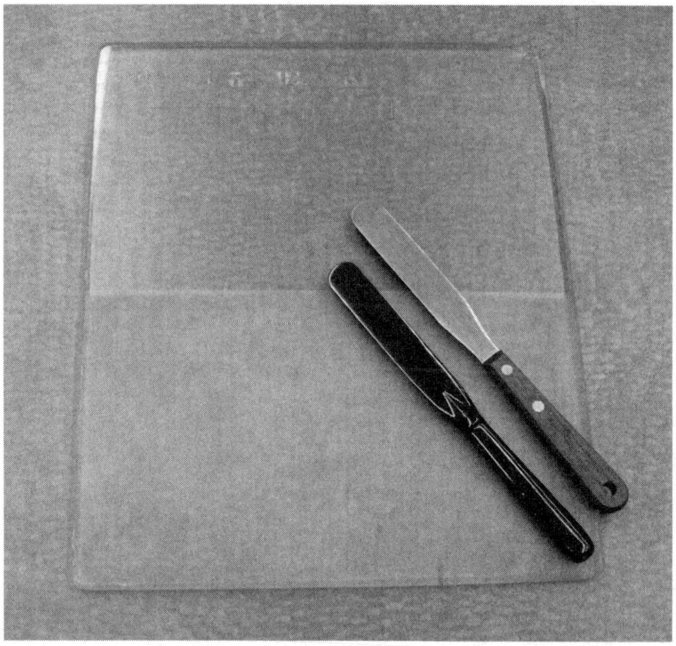

Figure 1–3. Ointment slab.

introducing drugs into the body. Medications are not beneficial to the patient until they reach the blood and are distributed to the body. IV medications are introduced directly into the blood and therefore have the most rapid onset of action. IV medications, therefore, have many benefits over oral medications, which have to be absorbed from the gastrointestinal tract, or IM medications, which have to be absorbed through the muscle mass. IV medications can be given to patients who are unconscious, uncooperative, nauseated, vomiting, or otherwise unable to take medications orally. Direct administration of IV medications into the blood also provides a predictable rate of administration. Certainly, IV medications have disadvantages, such as the risk of infection, the pain of the injection, and the immediate effect of the administration in the

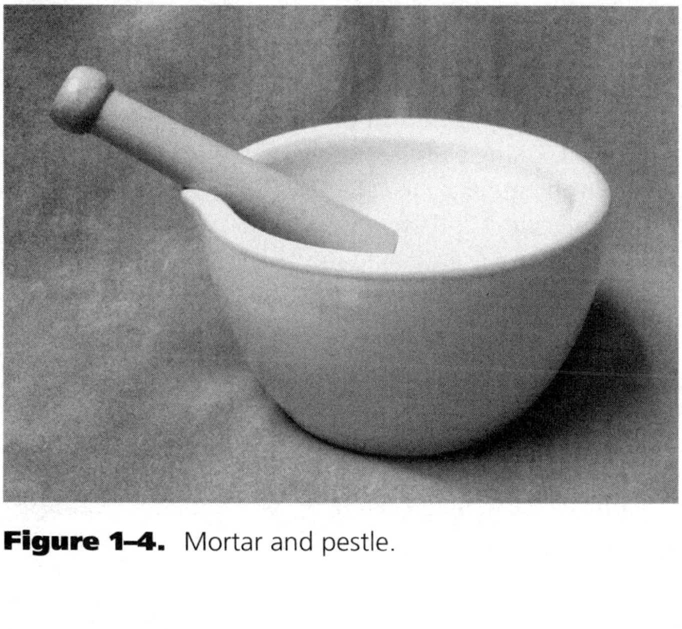

Figure 1–4. Mortar and pestle.

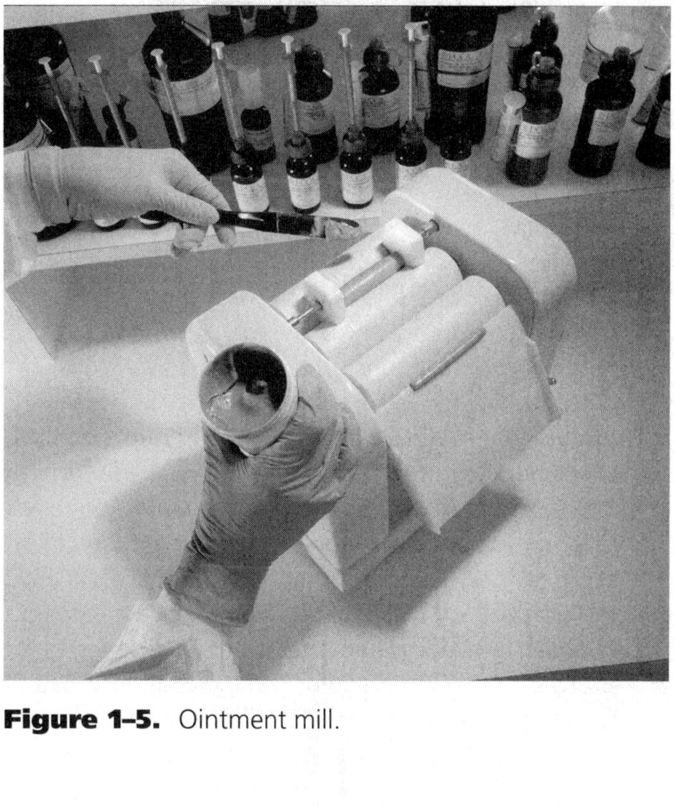

Figure 1–5. Ointment mill.

event of an error. Some medications are not suitable for IV administration because of their stability or absorptive properties.

Special training is required for personnel who prepare and administer sterile IV solutions. The process of preparing IV products using preset steps to ensure a sterile final product is known as *aseptic technique.* Basic aseptic technique should be used when handling parenteral dosage forms, as well as irrigations and ophthalmics (see Chapter 12 of the *Manual for Pharmacy Technicians,* Medication Dosage Forms and Routes of Administration).

Risks of IV Therapy

IV therapy offers a rapid, direct means of administering many life-saving drugs and fluids. A high percentage of IV therapy is administered without any problems, but there are some risks:

- *Infection*—Infections can result if a product contaminated with bacteria is infused into a patient. Because the IV bypasses the body's normal barrier system, bacteria reach the bloodstream directly. Bacteria can be introduced into products during preparation, administration, production, and through improper storage. The rate of infection or sepsis due to contaminated infusions has steadily decreased since health care practitioners and product manufacturers have implemented training and quality assurance programs. Despite these efforts, human touch contamination continues to be the most common source of IV-related contamination.
- *Air embolus*—The incidence of an air embolus is low because many solutions are administered using infusion pumps equipped with an alarm, called an *air-in-line alarm,* that sounds when air is in the IV line. Solutions infused by gravity do not need alarms because the infusion automatically stops when there is no more fluid for gravity to push through the IV line. Even when a bag runs dry, large amounts of air are not infused. In adults, 150 or 200 ml of air given quickly through an IV can result in harm. Infants and pediatric patients are adversely affected by a much lower amount of air. Filters are available on some IV sets, and they also stop air bubbles and add another measure of safety.
- *Bleeding*—IV therapy may cause bleeding. When the IV catheter is removed, bleeding may occur around the catheter site. If the patient has a condition that results in prolonged bleeding time, extra care and caution should be used, especially when removing the catheter.
- *Allergic reaction*—When a patient has an allergic reaction to a substance given parenterally, the reaction is usually more severe than if the same substance were given by another route (eg, by mouth, topically, or rectally). One reason for this is that substances given parenterally cannot be retrieved like substances given by other routes. For example, substances administered topically can easily be washed off, those given orally can be retrieved by inducing vomiting or by pumping the stomach, and those given rectally can be flushed out using an enema. When a drug that has caused allergic reactions in a large number of patients is given intravenously, the patient should be monitored closely. If the likelihood of an allergic reaction is especially high, a test dose (a small amount of the drug) may be given to see how the patient reacts.
- *Incompatibilities*—Some drugs are incompatible with other drugs, containers, or solutions. If an incompatibility exists, the drug may precipitate, be inactivated, or adhere to the container. These undesirable outcomes may be difficult to detect with the naked eye. A visual inspection of the final product should always be performed to observe any cloudiness, coring, or signs of irregularity. Solutions with known or detectable incompatibilities should not be administered to patients.
- *Extravasation*—Extravasation occurs when the IV catheter punctures and exits the vein under the skin, causing drugs to infuse or infiltrate into the tissue. Extravasation may happen when the catheter is being inserted or after it is in place if the extremity with the IV catheter is moved or flexed too much. Using a stiff-arm board to prevent excessive movement near the catheter site may help maintain regular flow and prevent extravasation and infiltration. Extravasation and infiltration can be painful and usually requires that the IV be restarted. Some drugs, such as certain chemotherapy agents, may cause severe tissue damage if they infiltrate the tissue. While there are medications to alleviate some of the effects of extravasation and hot and cold compresses to arrest progression, in some cases this tissue damage can be so severe that it requires surgery or even loss of the limb.

- *Particulate matter*—Particulate matter refers to unwanted particles present in parenteral products. Some examples of particulate matter are microscopic glass fragments, hair, lint or cotton fibers, cardboard fragments, undissolved drug particles, and fragments of rubber stoppers, known as cores. Particulate matter that is injected into the bloodstream can cause adverse effects. Improvements in the manufacturing processes have greatly reduced the presence of particulates in commercially available products. Care must be taken in the pharmacy so that particulate matter is not introduced into products. All products should be visually inspected for particulate matter before dispensing. Some institutions may use inline filters to help minimize the amount of particulate that reaches the patient.
- *Pyrogens*—Pyrogens, the by-products or remnants of bacteria, can cause reactions (eg, fever and chills) if injected in large enough amounts. Because a pyrogen can be present even after a solution has been sterilized, great care must be taken to ensure that these substances are not present.
- *Phlebitis*—Phlebitis, or irritation of the vein, may be caused by the IV catheter, the drug being administered (because of its chemical properties or its concentration), the location of the IV site, a fast rate of administration, or the presence of particulate matter. The patient usually feels pain or discomfort, often severe, along the path of the vein. Red streaking may also occur. If phlebitis is caused by a particular drug, further diluting the drug, then giving it more slowly, or giving it via an IV catheter placed in a vein with a higher, faster-moving volume of blood may be helpful.

Aseptic Preparation of Parenteral Products

As the use of parenteral therapy continues to expand, the need for well-controlled admixture preparation has also grown. Recognizing this need, many pharmacy departments have devoted increased resources to programs that ensure the aseptic preparation of sterile products. The following are the main elements on which these programs focus:

- Development and maintenance of good aseptic technique in the personnel who prepare and administer sterile products
- Development and maintenance of a sterile compounding area complete with sterilized equipment and supplies
- Development and maintenance of the skills needed to properly use an LAFW

Aseptic Technique

Aseptic technique is a means of manipulating sterile products without contaminating them. Proper use of an LAFW and strict aseptic technique are the most important factors in preventing the contamination of sterile products. Thorough training in the proper use of the LAFW and strict aseptic technique, followed by the development of conscientious work habits, is of utmost importance to any sterile products program.

Sterile Compounding Area, the Clean Room

Sterile parenteral solutions must be free of living microorganisms and relatively free of particles and pyrogens. Room air typically contains thousands of suspended particles per cubic foot, most of which are too small to be seen with the naked eye. These suspended particles include contaminants such as dust, pollen, smoke, and bacteria. Reducing the number of particles in the air improves the environment in which sterile products are prepared and can be done by following several practices.

A sterile compounding area's counters, work surfaces, and floors should be cleaned daily while walls, ceilings, and storage shelving should be cleaned monthly at a minimum. Segregated compounding areas must be separate from normal pharmacy operations, nonessential equipment, and other materials that produce particles. For example, the introduction of cardboard into the clean environment should be avoided. Traffic flow into a clean area should be minimized. Floors should be disinfected periodically, and trash should be removed frequently. Trashcans should be taken outside the IV room before pulling the trash from the container. This will minimize the creation of particulate matter and the risk of spills in the clean room. More sophisticated aspects of clean room design include special filtration or treatment systems for incoming air, ultraviolet irradiation, air-lock entry portals, sticky mats to remove particulates from shoes, and positive room air pressure to reduce contaminant entry from adjacent rooms or hallways. Clean rooms are often adjoined by a room, called an *anteroom,* that is used for nonaseptic activities related to the clean room operation, such as order processing, gowning, and stock storage.

Sterile products should be prepared in Class 100 environments, which means environments containing no more than 100 particles per cubic foot that are 0.5 micron or larger in size. LAFWs are frequently used to achieve a Class 100 environment.

Laminar Airflow Workbenches

The underlying principle of laminar airflow workbenches (LAFW) is that twice-filtered laminar layers of aseptic air continuously sweep the work area inside the hood to prevent the entry of contaminated room air. There are two common types of LAFW: horizontal flow and vertical flow.

Horizontal LAFW

LAFW that sweep filtered air from the back of the hood to the front are called horizontal LAFW (see Figure1-6). Horizontal flow workbenches use an electrical blower to draw contaminated room air through a prefilter. The prefilter, which is similar to a furnace filter, removes only gross contaminants and should be cleaned or replaced regularly. The prefiltered air is then pressurized to ensure that a consistent distribution of airflow is presented to the final filtering apparatus. The final filter constitutes the entire back portion of the hood's work area. This high efficiency particulate air, or HEPA, filter removes 99.97% of particles that are 0.3 micron or larger, thereby eliminating airborne microorganisms, which are usually 0.5 microns or larger.

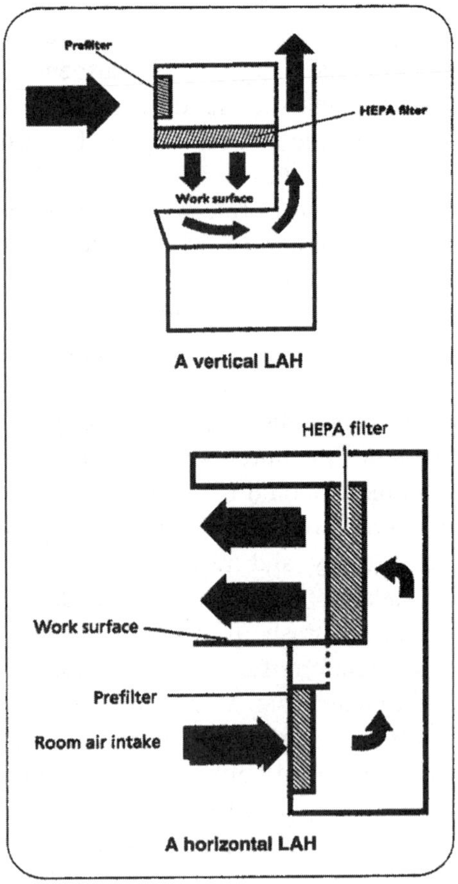

Figure 1-6. Horizontal and vertical laminar airflow workbench with the basic components labeled.

Vertical LAFW

Laminar flow workbenches with a vertical flow of filtered air are also available. In vertical LAFW, HEPA-filtered air emerges from the top and passes downward through the work area (see Figure 1-6). Because exposure to some antineoplastic (anticancer) drugs may be harmful, these drugs are usually prepared in vertical LAFW to minimize the risk of exposure to airborne drug particulates. The types of vertical laminar airflow hoods (LAH) used for the preparation of antineoplastics contain airflow within the hood and are referred to as biological safety cabinets (BSC).

The critical principle of using LAFW is that nothing must interrupt the flow of air between the HEPA filter and the sterile object. The space between the HEPA filter and the sterile object is known as the *critical area.* The introduction of a foreign object between a sterile object and the HEPA filter increases wind turbulence in the critical area and the possibility that contaminants from the foreign object may be carried onto the sterile work surface and thereby contaminate an injection port, needle, or syringe. To maintain sterility, nothing should pass behind a sterile object in a horizontal LAH or above a sterile object in a vertical LAFW.

Materials placed within the LAFW disturb the patterned flow of air blowing from the HEPA filter. The zone of turbulence created behind an object could potentially extend outside the hood, pulling or allowing contaminated room air into the aseptic working area. When laminar airflow is moving on all sides of an object, the zone of turbulence extends approximately three times the diameter of that object. When laminar airflow is not accessible to an object on all sides (for example, when placed adjacent to a vertical wall), the zone of turbulence may extend six times the diameter of the object. Working with objects at least 6 inches from the sides and front edge of the hood, without blocking air vents is therefore advisable to maintain unobstructed airflow between the HEPA filter and sterile objects. The hands should be positioned so that airflow in the critical area between the HEPA filter and sterile objects is not blocked.

The following are general principles for operating LAFWs properly:

- An LAFW should be positioned away from excess traffic, doors, air vents, or anything that could produce air currents capable of introducing contaminants into the hood.
- If an LAFW is turned off, nonfiltered, nonsterile air will occupy the LAFW work area. Therefore, when it is turned back on, it should be allowed to run for 15 to 30 minutes before it is used (manufacturer recommendations should be consulted for each hood). This time allows the LAFW to blow the nonsterile air out of the LAFW work area. Then the LAFW can be cleaned for use.
- Before using the LAFW, all its interior working surfaces should be cleaned with 70% isopropyl alcohol or another appropriate disinfecting agent and a clean, lint-free cloth. Cleaning should be performed from the HEPA filter in a side-to-side motion beginning in the rear of the hood and moving toward the front (in a horizontal LAFW) so contaminants are moved out of the hood. The hood should be cleaned often throughout the compounding period and when the work surface becomes dirty. Some materials are not soluble in alcohol and may initially require the use of water to be removed. After the water is applied, the surface should be cleaned with alcohol. Plexiglas sides, found on some types of LAFWs, should be cleaned with warm, soapy water rather than alcohol. Spray bottles of alcohol should not be used in the LAFW, and because they do not allow for the physical action of cleaning the hood, they can damage the HEPA filter, and they do not ensure that alcohol is applied to all areas of the surface to be cleaned. Alcohol should be allowed to dry to increase its effectiveness as a disinfectant.
- Nothing should be permitted to come in contact with the HEPA filter. This includes cleaning solution, aspirate from syringes, or glass from ampules. Ampules should not be opened directly toward the filter.
- Only objects essential to product preparation should be placed in the LAFW. Paper, pens, labels, or trays should not be placed in the hood.
- Jewelry should not be worn on the hands or wrists when working in the LAFW because it may introduce bacteria or particles into the clean work area.
- Actions such as talking and coughing should be directed away from the LAFW working area, and unnecessary motion within the hood should be avoided to minimize the turbulence of airflow.
- Smoking, eating, and drinking are prohibited in the aseptic environment.
- All aseptic manipulations should be performed at least 6 inches within the hood to prevent potential contamination caused by the closeness of the worker's body and backwash contamination resulting from turbulent air patterns developing where LAFW air meets room air.
- LAFWs should be tested by qualified personnel every 6 months, whenever the hood is moved, or if filter damage is suspected. Specific tests are used to certify airflow velocity and HEPA filter integrity.

Although the LAFW provides an aseptic environment, safe for the manipulation of sterile products, strict aseptic technique must be used in conjunction with proper hood operation. The use of the LAFW alone, without the observance of aseptic technique, cannot ensure product sterility.

Personal Attire

The first component of good aseptic technique is proper personal attire. Compounding personnel should remove personal outer garments, all cosmetics, and all hand, wrist, and other visible jewelry or piercings before entering the ante room or segregated compounding area. Clean room attire should include dedicated shoes or shoe covers, head and facial hair covers, and face masks/eye shields applied in this order to help reduce particulate or bacterial contamination. After hand washing as described below, clean garments, which are relatively particulate free, should be worn when preparing sterile products. Clean room attire will depend on institutional policies and often are related to the type of product being prepared. Many facilities provide clean scrub suits or gowns for this purpose. Scrub suits should not be worn home to ensure that no contaminants are transported home and that the process of cleaning the clothing does not introduce lint onto the low-lint clothing. In addition, suits should be covered up when leaving the pharmacy to minimize the contamination from areas such as the cafeteria.

Pop Quiz!

Work inside an LAFW must be done at least how many inches from the sides?

Handwashing

Touching sterile products while compounding is the most common source of contamination of pharmacy-prepared sterile products. Because the fingers harbor countless bacterial contaminants, proper hand washing is extremely important. Every entry into a sterile product should include scrubbing your hands, nails, wrists, and forearms to elbows thoroughly for at least 30 seconds with a brush, warm water, and appropriate bactericidal soap before performing aseptic manipulations. Dry hands completely, using either lint-free disposable towels or an electronic hand dryer.

Gloving

After appropriate hand washing is complete and attire is put on, antiseptic hand cleansing should be performed using a waterless, alcohol-based surgical hand scrub just prior to the last item worn before compounding begins, sterile gloves. Sterile gloves are only sterile until they touch something unsterile or until they are torn and allow bacteria from the hands to enter the work area. For example, if it becomes necessary to scratch or touch the face while wearing gloves, they will need to be changed. For these reasons, always wash your bare hands thoroughly as noted above, before unwrapping and putting on the gloves. Occasionally, workers develop allergies to latex as a result of repeated use of latex gloves. As a result, many institutions have now turned to using only non-latex gloves.

Equipment and Supplies

Another important factor in aseptic preparation of sterile products is the correct use of appropriate sterile equipment and supplies, including syringes and needles.

Syringes

Syringes are made of either glass or plastic. Most drugs are more stable in glass, so glass syringes are most often used when medication is to be stored in the syringe for an extended period. Some medications may react with the

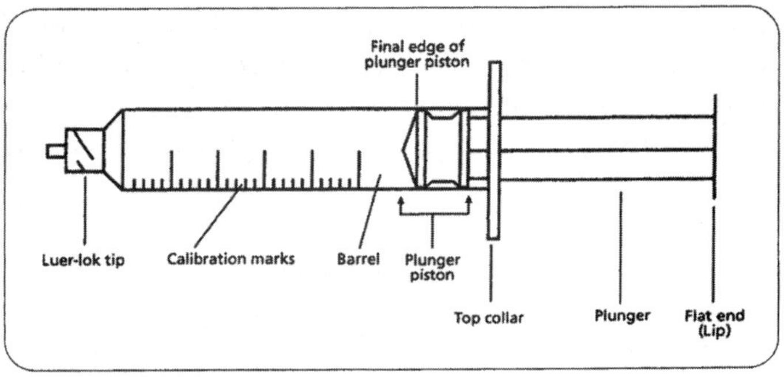

Figure 1-7. A syringe with the basic components labeled.

plastics in the syringe, which would alter the potency or stability of the final product. Disposable plastic syringes are most frequently used in preparing sterile products because they are cheaper, durable, and are in contact with substances only for a short time. This minimizes the potential for incompatibility with the plastic itself.

Syringes are composed of a barrel and plunger (see Figure 1-7). The plunger, which fits inside the barrel, has a flat disk or lip at one end and a rubber piston at the other. The top collar of the barrel prevents the syringe from slipping during manipulation; the tip is where the needle attaches. To maintain sterility of the product, the syringe tip or the plunger should not be touched. Many syringes have a locking mechanism at the tip, such as the Luer-lock, which secures the needle within a threaded ring. Some syringes, such as slip-tip syringes, do not have a locking mechanism. In this case, friction holds the needle on the syringe.

Syringes are available in numerous sizes, ranging from 0.5 to 60 milliliters (ml). Calibration marks on syringes represent different increments of capacity, depending on the size of the syringe. Usually, the larger the syringe capacity, the larger the interval between calibration lines. For example, each line on a 10 ml syringes represents 0.2 ml, but on a 30 ml syringe, each line represents 1 ml.

To maximize accuracy, the smallest syringe that can hold a desired amount of solution should be used. Syringes are accurate to one-half of the smallest increment marking on the barrel. For example, a 10 ml syringe with 0.2 ml markings is accurate to 0.1 ml and can be used to measure 3.1 ml accurately. A 30 ml syringe with 1 ml markings, however, is only accurate to 0.5 ml and should not be used to measure a volume of 3.1 ml. Ideally, the volume of solution should only take up one-half to two-thirds of the syringe capacity. This avoids inadvertent touch contamination when the syringe plunger is pulled all the way back.

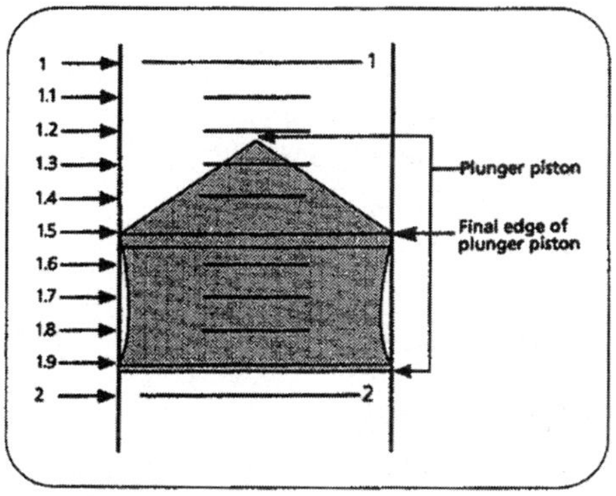

Figure 1-8. A close-up of a syringe showing how to measure 1.5 ml. Note that the final edge of the plunger piston is used to make the measurement.

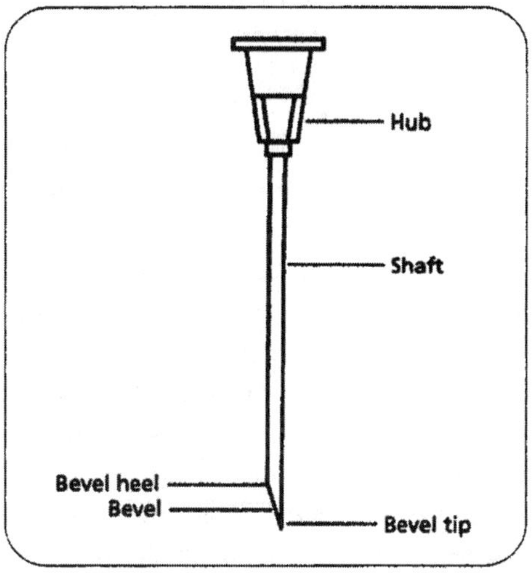

Figure 1-9. A needle with the basic components labeled.

When measuring with a syringe, the final edge (closest to the tip of the syringe) of the plunger piston, which comes in contact with the syringe barrel, should be lined up with the calibration mark on the barrel that corresponds to the volume desired (see Figure 1-8).

Syringes are sent from the manufacturer assembled and individually packaged in paper overwraps or plastic covers. The sterility of the contents is guaranteed as long as the outer package remains intact. Therefore, packages should be inspected, and any that are damaged should be discarded. The syringe package should be opened within the LAH to maintain sterility. The wrapper should be peeled apart, not ripped or torn. To minimize particulate contamination, discarded packaging or unopened syringes should not be placed on the LAFW work surface.

Syringes may come from the manufacturer with a needle attached or with a protective cover over the syringe tip. The syringe tip protector should be left in place until it is time to attach the needle. For attaching needles to Luer-lock-type syringes, a quarter turn is usually sufficient to secure the needle to the syringe.

Needles

Like syringes, needles are commercially available in many sizes. Sizes are described by two numbers: gauge and length. The gauge of the needle corresponds to the diameter of its bore, which is the diameter of the inside of the shaft. The larger the gauge, the smaller the needle bore. For example, the smallest needles have a gauge of 27, whereas the largest needles have a gauge of 13. The length of a needle shaft is measured in inches and usually ranges from 3/8 to 3 1/2 inches.

The components of a simple needle are the shaft and the hub (see Figure 1-9). The hub attaches the needle to the syringe and is often color-coded to correspond to a specific gauge. The tip of the needle shaft is slanted to form a point. The slant is called the *bevel,* and the point is called the *bevel tip.* The opposite end of the slant is called the *bevel heel.*

Needles are sent from the manufacturer individually packaged in paper or plastic overwraps with a protective cover over the needle shaft. This guarantees the sterility as long as the package remains intact. Damaged packages should be discarded.

No part of the needle itself should be touched. Needles should be manipulated by their overwrap and protective covers only. The protective cover should be left in place until the needle or syringe is ready to be used. A needle shaft is usually metal and is lubricated with a sterile silicone coating so latex vial tops can be penetrated smoothly and easily. For this reason, needles should never be swabbed with alcohol.

Some needles are designed for special purposes and therefore have unique characteristics. For example, needles designed for batch filling have built-in vents (vented needles) to avoid the need to release pressure that might form in the vial. Another example is needles with built-in filters, meant to be used with products requiring filtering, such as drugs removed from a glass ampule.

Drug Additive Containers

Injectable medication additives may be supplied in an ampule, vial, or prefilled syringe. Each requires a different technique to withdraw medication and place it in the final dosage form.

Vials

Medication vials are glass or plastic containers with a rubber stopper secured to the top, usually by an aluminum cover. Vials differ from ampules in that they are used to hold both powders and liquids. The rubber stopper is usually protected by a flip-top plastic cap or aluminum cover.

Protective covers do not guarantee sterility of the rubber stopper. Therefore, before the stopper is penetrated, it must be swabbed with 70% isopropyl alcohol and allowed to dry. The correct swabbing technique is to make several firm strokes in the same direction over the rubber closure, always using a clean swab.

Vials are closed-system containers, because air or fluid cannot pass freely in or out of them. In most cases, air pressure inside the vial is similar to that of room air. In order to prevent the formation of a vacuum inside the vial (less pressure inside the vial than room air), the pressure should be normalized by first injecting a volume of air equal to the volume of fluid that is going to be withdrawn, into the vial. This step should not be done with drugs that produce gas when they are reconstituted, such as ceftazidime, or with cytotoxic medications.

Ampules

Ampules are composed entirely of glass and, once broken (ie, opened), become open-system containers (Figure 1-10). Because air or fluid may now pass freely in and out of the container (no vacuum effect), it is not necessary to replace the volume of fluid to be withdrawn with air.

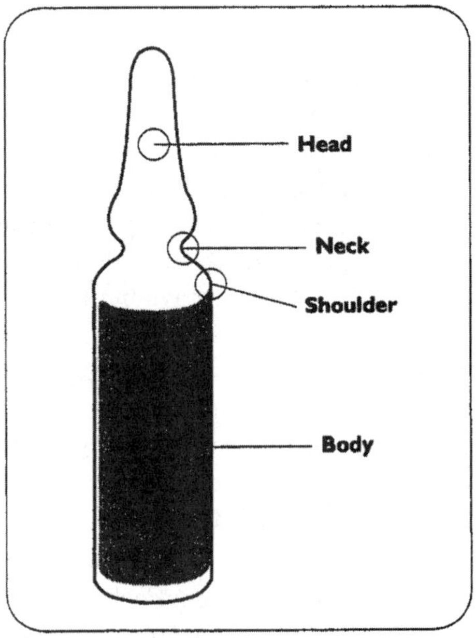

Figure 1-10. An ampule with the basic components.

To open an ampule, the head must be broken from the body of the ampule. To make the break properly, the ampule neck is cleansed with an alcohol swab and the swab should be left in place. This swab can prevent accidental cuts to the fingers as well as shattering of glass particles and aerosolized drug.

Automated Compounding Sterile Product Filling Equipment

Although hospitals and regulatory agencies have strict guidelines that must be followed, including rigorous training and competencies, the technical complexity of sterile product preparation lends itself to inconsistency among employees. Additionally, compounded sterile products create potentially challenging situations for pharmacists to verify product preparation accuracy. Automation can eliminate sources of preparation errors inherent to human factors; this technology ensures proper handling, and accurate and sterile preparation of the IV product.

? Pop Quiz!

What kind of needle is used to withdraw liquid from an ampule?

Labeling

Once an IV admixture or other sterile product is compounded, it should be properly labeled with the following information:

1. Patient name, identification number, and room number (if applicable)
2. Bottle or bag sequence number, when appropriate
3. Name and amount of drug(s) added
4. Name and volume of admixture solution
5. Approximate final total volume of the admixture, when applicable
6. Prescribed flow rate (in milliliters per hour)
7. Date and time of scheduled administration
8. Date and time of preparation
9. Expiration date
10. Initials of person who prepared and person who checked the IV admixture
11. Auxiliary labeling—supplemental instructions and precautions

Many labels also now contain a bar code that contains information regarding the medication, the patient, and the anticipated administration. These are generated by the pharmacy computer to reduce the frequency of medication administration errors. Each product should also include an expiration date, beyond which it should not be used.

Preparation and Handling of Cytotoxic and Hazardous Drugs

Some medications can be hazardous to those who touch or inhale them. Because hazardous drugs initially involved drugs used to treat cancer, the terms antineoplastic and chemotherapeutic were used to describe them.

Preparation of these agents requires special procedures for labeling, storage, and transport. Use of protective clothing, BSCs, and special handling of spills and waste are also important. Special techniques related to the actual administration of these products to patients are not covered here. Additional information is available from ASHP in the form of a *Technical Assistance Bulletin on Handling of Cytotoxic and Hazardous Drugs.*

Protective Apparel

There is no substitute for good technique, but protective apparel is another fundamental element in protecting personnel who handle or prepare hazardous drugs.

Most procedures require the use of disposable coveralls or a solid front gown. These garments should be made of low-permeability, lint-free fabric. They must have long sleeves and tight-fitting elastic or knit cuffs. They should not be worn outside the work area and should be changed immediately if contaminated. Shoe and hair covers may also be required, depending on the institution's policies.

Wearing gloves is essential when working with hazardous drugs. Wash hands thoroughly before putting on the gloves and after removing them. Use good quality, disposable, powder-free latex gloves, such as surgical latex. These gloves are preferred because of their fit, elasticity, and tactile sensation. If only powdered gloves are available, wash powder off before beginning to work. Non-latex gloves are also available for those with an allergy to latex. If two pairs are needed, tuck one pair under the cuffs of the gown and place the second pair over the cuff. If an outer glove becomes contaminated, change it immediately. Change both the inner and the outer gloves immediately if the outer glove becomes torn, punctured, or heavily contaminated. If only one pair is worn, tuck the glove under or over the gown cuff so that the skin is not exposed.

Biological Safety Cabinets

One of the most important pieces of equipment for handling hazardous drugs safely is the **Biological Safety Cabinet (BSC).** A BSC is a type of vertical LAFW that is designed to protect workers from exposure as well as to help maintain product sterility during preparation. BSCs must meet standards set by the National Sanitation Foundation (NSF Standard 49). Do not use horizontal LAFWs to prepare hazardous drugs. BSCs must be operated continuously, 24 hours per day, and they should be inspected and certified by qualified personnel every 6 months.

Preparing Hazardous Drugs

Before technicians handle a cytotoxic or other hazardous drug, they must demonstrate proper manipulative technique and use of protective equipment and materials.

Drug Information

Pharmacy technicians are challenged with drug information questions frequently throughout the workday and are called upon to become knowledgeable about the handling, availability, and uses of medications. A basic knowledge of the resources available will make the technician more resourceful and better able to assist the pharmacist with certain drug information requests. Pharmacy reference books and electronic media (including the Internet) that are available in all practice settings often hold answers to typical day-to-day practice-related questions. Before responding to a drug information question, technicians must clearly differentiate questions that fall within their scope of practice from those that must be answered only by a pharmacist.

Technicians should identify themselves as pharmacy technicians so the person asking the question will know the type of information that may appropriately be conveyed. If there is any doubt about the nature of the question, the technician should defer the question to the pharmacist. It is important for the technician to learn who the person initiating the request is and to obtain the necessary contact information (phone, fax, pager, etc.) in case the person needs to be called back. The search for and response to drug information requests will be different depending on who is requesting the information. Knowing information

Table 1-1. Classifications of Drug Information Questions

Question Classification	Examples
General Drug Information	What is the brand name of warfarin? Do Naprosyn and Aleve contain the same active ingredient? Who manufactures Enbrel? Is Prilosec available as a generic? Is it a prescription or over-the-counter (OTC) product?
Availability and Cost	What dosage forms of Imitrex are available in your pharmacy? Is Zoloft available as a liquid? If so, what size and concentration is available? What are the prices of Adalat CC and Procardia XL? How long is the shortage of albumin expected to last?
Storage and Stability	Should Lovenox be stored in the refrigerator? How long is a flu shot stable after it is drawn up in a syringe?
Calculations	How many milliliters are in an ounce?
Preparation	How should ampicillin be reconstituted?
Pharmacy Law	In what controlled substance schedule is zolpidem (Ambien)? Can Tiazac be substituted for Cardizem CD (is it AB rated)? How many times can a prescription be transferred from one store to another?
Miscellaneous	Where can I find the phone number for Sanofi Aventis? When will the patent for Lipitor expire? Where can I get more Lovenox teaching kits? Where can I find the Vaccine Information Sheet for the influenza vaccine?

about the requestor, their training, and their knowledge of the subject will have an impact on what the final response will be and how it will be given. Obtaining background information will help to determine what the needs of the requestor are and will make the search for information more efficient. Background information is especially important to determine if the question pertains to a specific patient or if it is a question that requires interpretation, and therefore the expertise of a pharmacist. The urgency of the request and the extent of the information needed should also be determined so an appropriate amount of time is allotted to answer the request. Classifying the type of request helps to narrow the search and makes the search process more efficient. Table 1-1 lists common types of questions that technicians may get, with examples of each. Technicians should not interpret a patient-specific question or provide information that may require professional judgment. A simply stated question can actually be a complex patient-specific situation. The pharmacist has to find out more about the patient's specific problems and apply clinical judgment to answer the question appropriately. Many times, the person requesting the information may indirectly be asking for a pharmacist's point of view or interpretation of a situation, and may thus require an in-depth analysis and recommendation from the pharmacist. Attempting to interpret or answer such a question could result in miscommunication and delivery of inaccurate information. Both scenarios could be potentially harmful to the patient. Examples of questions that require a pharmacist's interpretation and that should not be answered by a technician are provided in Table 1-2.

Conducting the Search: Choosing the Right References

The key to answering questions quickly and accurately is knowing where the necessary information is likely to be found. The first step is to consult tertiary references, then secondary references, and finally primary references.

Tertiary references are general references that present documented information in a condensed and compact format. They include textbooks; compendia (eg, *American Hospital Formulary Service, Drug Information (AHFS DI), Drug Facts and Comparisons*); computerized systems such as Micromedex® Clinical Information System; review articles; and much of the information found on the Internet. Tertiary references are easy to use, convenient, readily accessible, concise, and compact. Disadvantages of tertiary references are that information may not be timely, the information could contain errors, and tertiary references may not offer enough information on a specific topic because of space restrictions.

Table 1–2. Drug Information Questions Appropriate for Pharmacists

Question Classification	Examples	Rationale
Identification and Availability	What is paracetamol and what is its U.S. equivalent?	Although it is appropriate for a technician to obtain technical information about availability (eg, anticipated length/reasons for a shortage), questions that require clinical knowledge, such as therapeutic alternatives, must be answered by a pharmacist
Allergies	Which narcotic is safe to use in a patient with a codeine allergy?	For allergy questions, the pharmacist must obtain more patient-specific information, such as a description of the allergy and the condition being treated. Clinical judgment is required.
Dosing and Administration	What is the usual dose of propranolol? How long should ciprofloxacin be given for a urinary tract infection? What is the best way to give gentamicin IV?	Answers to dosing and administration questions depend on many factors, especially the indication for use and patient-specific information (eg, age, weight, and kidney and liver function).
Compatibility	Is Primaxin compatible with dopamine?	More information is needed (eg, doses, concentrations, fluids, and type of IV lines), and a pharmacist must interpret information found in a reference and apply it to the situation.
Drug Interactions	Is it OK to take aspirin with warfarin?	Drug interaction questions are complex and require patient-specific information and interpretation by a pharmacist in order to apply the significance of a potential interaction to a specific patient.
Side Effects	What are the side effects of Lexapro? Can Celebrex cause renal failure?	Package inserts and textbooks provide lists of side effects that are often difficult to interpret and convey. Also, a pharmacist must interpret whether the request is being made because an adverse event is suspected with one or more medications.
Pregnancy and Lactation	Is albuterol safe to use in pregnancy? Can I get a flu shot if I am breastfeeding?	Pregnancy and lactation questions are complicated because more information is needed about the patient, the stage of pregnancy, and/or age of the infant. A pharmacist must interpret the findings and apply them to the specific situation.
Therapeutic Use	Has clonidine been used to treat opiate withdrawal?	The use of drugs for non-FDA approved uses often requires evaluation and interpretation of the literature and clinical judgment.

Secondary references include indexing systems such as Medline that provide a list of journal articles on the topic that is being researched. Secondary systems are used when new or very up-to-date information is required or when no information can be found in tertiary references.

Primary references are original research articles published in scientific journals, such as the *American Journal of Health-System Pharmacy (AJHP)* or the *Journal of the American Pharmacists Association (JAPhA)*.

Other resources include pharmaceutical manufacturers and specialized drug and poison information centers.

If the information cannot be found in a tertiary reference, then the technician should consult a pharmacist, who may advise an alternative search strategy or consult a secondary reference. If time permits, the technician should consult as many resources as possible and compare information among resources.

Common References

Technicians should familiarize themselves with the references in their practice settings to determine which sources best fit their needs. Using a systematic approach when faced with a drug information question will aid in understanding the nature of the request, obtaining pertinent background information, and answering the question. Numerous resources are available to assist with answering drug information requests. Becoming familiar with common resources will make the search process more efficient. It is critical for pharmacy technicians to be able to differentiate between basic drug information questions that they can answer and questions that require clinical

Table 1-3. Common Drug Information Requests and Reference Sources

Type of Information Needed	References Likely to Have the Information
Product Availability dosage form product strength brand and generic name manufacturer indication	Facts & Comparisons Drug Information Handbook Internet PDR Micromedex Clinical Pharmacology RedBook (not indication) USPDI Pharmaceutical Manufacturer
Product Identification dosage form product strength brand and generic name manufacturer colored photographs of tablets/capsules	Facts & Comparisons PDR Clinical Pharmacology USPDI Micromedex
Drug Uses FDA-approved indications other uses of the agent	AHFS Clinical Pharmacology Facts & Comparisons Drug Information Handbook PDR (FDA-approved indications only) Micromedex USPDI
Drug Monographs general drug information pharmacology indications and uses drug interactions admixture information doses adverse effects drug interactions	AHFS Clinical Pharmacology Facts & Comparisons Drug Information Handbook Micromedex PDR USPDI
Injectable Drug Compatibility/Stability Information drug diluent and solution compatibilities drug compatibility conditions for handling and storing products (ie, glass vs. plastic container, protection from light, filters, refrigeration, expiration, etc.)	AHFS King's Guide Trissel's Handbook on Injectable Drugs Package inserts PDR Micromedex
Preparation	AHFS King's Guide Trissel's Handbook on Injectable Drugs Micromedex Package inserts PDR
Calculations	Drug Information Handbook Micromedex
Hazardous Chemicals and Drugs specifies hazards of the chemicals or drugs used at the worksite guidelines for their safe use recommendations to treat or clean up an exposure	Material Safety Data Sheets Micromedex
Pharmacy Law Generic substitution (bioequivalence) Federal regulations regarding handling and dispensing	USPDI Volume III Orange Book
Patient Information	Clinical Pharmacology Facts & Comparisons Internet Lexi-Comp MedlinePlus Micromedex Patient package inserts, Medication Guides USPDI Volume I

judgment, and therefore should be answered by a pharmacist. The references described in the next few sections are summarized in Table 1-3 with examples of the types of information one might find in each.

General Drug Information

Drug Facts and Comparisons (a part of Wolters Kluwers Health) is easy to use and available in regularly updated print and electronic versions. It is a comprehensive general drug information reference that provides complete drug monographs. It is organized by therapeutic class (eg, antihistamines, topicals) and includes tables that allow quick comparisons of drugs within the same class.

United States Pharmacopeia Drug Information (*USPDI,* published by Thomson) is a three-volume set that provides medication information for health care professionals (Volume I) and patients (Volume II). The third volume (*Approved Drug Products and Legal Requirements*) provides information on laws affecting pharmacy practice.

The Physicians' Desk Reference (*PDR,* published by Thomson Medical Economics) contains manufacturers' package inserts. A package insert is a manufacturer's product information sheet that provides general drug information, such as how the drug works, indications, adverse effects, drug interactions, dosage forms, stability, and dosing information. The *PDR* is not comprehensive and contains information only on select brand name drugs. The information is written by the manufacturer and approved by the FDA. It contains only information about FDA-approved uses of the drug and does not provide information comparing that drug with similar medications. Therefore, using the *PDR* to compare products is not as straightforward as using other reference books.

American Hospital Formulary Service Drug Information (*AHFS DI,* published by the American Society of Health-System Pharmacists, ASHP) is a detailed, comprehensive, general drug information reference. This textbook provides complete drug monographs that are organized by therapeutic class (eg, anti-infectives, cardiovascular). It provides detailed information about the use of a drug, its side effects, dosing considerations, and so on, and its coverage is not limited to FDA-approved uses of medications. It is especially useful for preparation and administration instructions for injectable products.

Lexi-Comp's Drug Information Handbook and Drug Information Handbook for the Allied Health Professional (published by Lexi-Comp) are handbooks containing general drug information monographs. They are widely used because they are quick, convenient, and easy to use. The *Drug Information Handbook* is alphabetically organized in dictionary format according to generic name. The *Drug Information Handbook for the Allied Health Professional* is not as comprehensive as the *Drug Information Handbook,* but it may be appealing to technicians because it allows quick access to basic data on the most frequently used medications. Both publications contain extensive appendixes with helpful charts, abbreviations, measurements, and conversions.

Mosby's Drug Consult (published by Elsevier Science) is a comprehensive general drug information reference. It provides complete drug monographs that are organized alphabetically by generic drug names. This textbook is more comprehensive than the *PDR.* A key feature is its indexing system, which allows identification of all drugs within a therapeutic class, schedules of controlled substances, pregnancy categories, and so on.

American Drug Index (published by Facts and Comparisons) is an alphabetical listing of drugs with brief information on each agent, including drug name (generic, brand, chemical name), manufacturer, dosage form, strength and packaging information, and general uses (eg, general anesthetic, narcotic, antitussive). It also contains pharmaceutical manufacturers' phone numbers and addresses, weight and measuring conversions, and a list of drugs that should not be crushed. Its extensive cross-indexing is useful to quickly identify a brand or generic product or determine product availability information.

Micromedex® Healthcare Series is a comprehensive reference system that is accessed electronically via CD-ROM, Internet, or personal digital assistant (PDA). Depending on the subscription, it contains comprehensive drug information, poison information, foreign drug information, tablet and capsule identification, disease and trauma information, herbal information, stability information, compatibility information, pregnancy information, patient information, and more.

Specialty References

Availability/Cost

Red Book (published by Medical Economics) contains up-to-date product information and prices for prescription drugs, over-the-counter products, and medical supplies. It contains NDC numbers for all products, available packaging, and therapeutic equivalence ratings (according to the FDA's *Orange Book*). It has a comprehensive listing of manufacturers, wholesalers, and third-party administrator directories. There are sections with other useful practical information, such as lists of sugar-, lactose-, galactose-, and alcohol-free products; sulfite-containing products; medications that should not be crushed; and color photographs of many prescription and over-the-counter products.

Compatibility and Stability

Trissel's Handbook on Injectable Drugs (published by American Society of Health-System Pharmacists, ASHP) is a textbook often used in hospital and home health care pharmacies. It focuses solely on injectable medications. Information includes data on the solubility, compatibility, and stability of many different medications. Specifically, this handbook is useful to determine when two medications may be safely mixed together in an IV bag, a syringe, or at a Y-site on an administration set. This reference also addresses special handling requirements of certain agents (glass vs. plastic containers, light restrictions, filters, refrigeration requirements, expiration, etc.).

King Guide to Parenteral Admixtures (published by King Guide Publications, Inc.) is another reference that is useful for compatibility and stability of injectable medications.

Extended Stability of Parenteral Drugs

Extended Stability of Parenteral Drugs (published by American Society of Health-System Pharmacists, ASHP) contains stability data of injectable drugs that extends beyond 24 hours. The reference is intended for use by alternate site infusion practices, such as home infusion.

Compounding

USP Pharmacist's Pharmacopeia (published by U.S. Pharmacopeia) is a reference that includes the official standards and procedures to ensure the strength, quality and purity of sterile and non-sterile compounded preparations. The individual drug monographs contain information on compounding, packaging, labeling, and storage of pharmaceuticals. The reference also includes information on veterinary compounding and food ingredients, colorings, preservatives, and flavorings. It is a useful resource for pharmacy compounding because it provides information on legal requirements and laws that apply to compounding practices, as well as articles on the basics of compounding.

Trissel's Stability of Compounded Formulations (published by the American Pharmacists Association, APhA) summarizes formulation and stability studies that are published for compounded formulations. Its drug monographs provide guidance for preparing the products as well as expiration dating, proper storage, and repackaging.

Herbal Medications and Dietary Supplements

Natural Medicines Comprehensive Database (published by Therapeutic Research Faculty) is a commonly used reference for natural medicines, including herbals and dietary supplements. Individual monographs list the name of the product, its common and scientific names, uses, safety, effectiveness, dosage and interactions with drugs, foods, labs, or diseases/conditions. It is available in both print and electronic forms.

Miscellaneous References

Material Safety Data Sheets (MSDS) are information sheets provided by manufacturers for chemicals or drugs that may be hazardous in the workplace. The primary purpose of the MSDS is to provide information about the specific hazards of the chemicals or drugs (ie, to describe acute and chronic health effects), guidelines for their safe use, and recommendations to treat an exposure or clean up a spill.

Drug Information and Poison Control Centers

Formal Drug Information Centers are another source of drug information. The centers throughout the country vary in the types of services they provide, but most centers provide drug information for health-care professionals, assist with formulary management, and train pharmacy students, residents, and pharmacists. Some centers provide drug information for consumers as well.

The Internet

The technician must take care to ensure that the information is current and up-to-date, and that it is accurate and from a reputable source. Generally, Web sites that are sponsored by the government, pharmacy and medical organizations, and medical centers are the most reputable. Table 1-4 lists useful Web sites for drug information and a brief description of what each site contains.

Pop Quiz!

Give an example of a comprehensive tertiary reference.

Table 1-4. Useful Web Sites for Obtaining Drug Information

Web site	Address	Description
Food and Drug Administration	www.fda.gov	Home page for the FDA; contains numerous useful links for both consumers and health-care professionals.
FDA Center for Drug Evaluation and Research (CDER)	www.fda.gov/cder	Contains links for consumers and health-care professionals regarding drug information, such as new drug approvals, drug shortages, safety information, and generic drug bioequivalence (Orange Book).
Drugs@FDA	www.accessdata.fda.gov/scripts/cder/drugsatfda/index.cfm	Contains information about FDA-approved drugs. Users can find package labeling information, generic drug products for brand name products, patient information (including Medication Guides), and review the approval history of drugs.
Centers for Disease Control and Prevention (CDC)	www.cdc.gov	Home page for the CDC; contains information about diseases, health topics, vaccines, traveler's health, bioterrorism, etc.
CDC Vaccine Information Statements	www.cdc.gov/vaccines/pubs/vis/default.htm	Link to Vaccine Information Statements that explain the benefits and risks of vaccines.
National Institutes for Health (NIH)	www.nih.gov	Home page for the NIH; contains information about health topics, clinical trials, and the various divisions of the NIH.
National Library of Medicine / Medline/ PubMed and MedlinePlus	www.nlm.nih.gov	Home page for the U.S. National Library of Medicine. Links to Medline Plus (health information for consumers) and Medline/PubMed (references and abstracts from biomedical journals).
American Society of Health-System Pharmacists (ASHP)	www.ashp.org	Home page for ASHP; contains news related to health-system pharmacy and many helpful links for pharmacy professionals.
ASHP Drug Shortages Resource Center	www.ashp.org/shortage	Up-to-date information on current drug shortages, including which products are affected and why, the anticipated time to resolution, and alternatives.
ASHP Consumer Drug Information	www.safemedication.com	Reputable Web site for patient medication information.
American Pharmacists Association (APhA)	www.pharmacist.com	Home page for APhA; contains news related to pharmacy and many helpful links for pharmacy professionals.
Institute for Safe Medication Practices (ISMP)	www.ismp.org	Homepage for the ISMP; contains medication error alerts, a section for reporting, products available for purchase, and medication error prevention strategies.
Virtual Library Pharmacy	www.pharmacy.org	Contains links to pharmacy associations, pharmaceutical manufacturers, governmental sites, hospitals, journals and books, and more.

Self-Assessment Questions

1. Abbreviations are generally considered to be unsafe and should therefore never be used in prescriptions.
   a. True
   b. False
2. The first step in receiving either a prescription or a medication order is to verify that all necessary information is present, although this information may vary depending on the pharmacy site (outpatient versus inpatient).
   a. True
   b. False
3. The abbreviation for "before meals" is
   a. a.a.
   b. hs
   c. pc
   d. ac
4. Which piece of information is critical in an ambulatory pharmacy environment when filling a prescription, but is often not known by the pharmacy in a hospital?
   a. patient's allergies
   b. name of the ordered drug
   c. dose of the ordered drug
   d. patient's insurance information
   e. name of the doctor
5. Every state's laws regarding prescription transfer are the same.
   a. True
   b. False
6. The first set of numbers in an NDC number signify
   a. the package size
   b. the specific product
   c. the manufacturer
   d. the schedule of the controlled substance
7. At the Point of Sale the patient's signature is required
   a. when they receive the HIPAA information
   b. when they receive a Patient Information Sheet
   c. by some third Party Companies when the patient receives the prescription
   d. in some states when they refuse counseling
   e. all the above
   f. a, c, and d only
8. Examples of drugs with REMS include clozapine, thalidomide, and
   a. isotretinoin and dofetilide
   b. isotretinoin and sildenafil
   c. alosetron and methadone
   d. sildenafil and tadalafil
9. Parenteral administration refers to drugs
   a. given by mouth
   b. administered only intravenously
   c. administered intravenously and intramuscularly
   d. given only subcutaneously
10. Which of the following is a possible risk associated with IV therapy?
    a. infection
    b. bleeding
    c. air embolus
    d. incompatibilities
    e. all of the above
11. Which of the following is false regarding the use of a Laminar Airflow Workbench (LAFW)?
    a. Hoods should be allowed to run for 15–30 minutes before use if they are not left on continuously.
    b. All compounding should be done at least 3 inches from the front edge of the hood.
    c. Only essential objects should be taken into the hood.
    d. Jewelry should not be worn on the hands or wrists when working in the hood.
    e. Actions such as talking or coughing should be directed from the LAFW work area.
12. Clean room attire should include
    a. shoe covers
    b. head covers
    c. facial hair covers
    d. face mask
    e. sterile gloves
    f. all the above

Self-Assessment Questions

13. Vials differ from ampoules in that they are used to hold both liquids and powders.
    a. True
    b. False
14. A ____ is the most important piece of equipment for handling and preparing hazardous drugs safely.
    a. LAFW
    b. BSC
    c. latex gloves
    d. automated compounder
15. Which reference is important in describing good compounding practices for technicians?
    a. Lexi-Comp's *Drug Information Handbook for the Allied Health Professional*
    b. Micromedex
    c. Package inserts
    d. *PDR*
    e. *USP 27*
16. Which question can a pharmacy technician answer?
    a. When will the shortage of methylprednisolone be over?
    b. How much acetaminophen should I give my 2 month old infant?
    c. Can propranolol make me dizzy?
    d. Does simvastatin interact with grapefruit juice?
    e. What should I substitute for morphine if my patient is allergic?
17. Which reference has the best information about IV compatibility?
    a. *American Drug Index*
    b. *PDR*
    c. *Drug Facts and Comparisons*
    d. Package inserts
    e. *Handbook on Injectable Drugs*
18. *Drug Facts and Comparisons* is considered a(n)
    a. tertiary general drug reference
    b. primary general drug reference
    c. specialty drug reference that includes only FDA approved drugs
19. The valid DEA number for Dr. Terry L Jones would be
    a. AT 4326915
    b. AJ 2178944
    c. AT 2178946
    d. AJ 432910
20. The NDC number for a product on the package label is 0536-3922-01. Which NDC number listed below would be in the proper form for this drug for remittance to a third party payer?
    a. 0536-3922-01
    b. 05363992201
    c. 00536-3922-01
    d. 05360-3922-01

Self-Assessment Answers

1. b
2. a
3. c
4. d
5. b
6. c
7. f
8. a
9. c
10. e
11. b
12. f
13. a
14. b
15. e
16. a
17. e
18. a
19. b
20. c

Chapter 2

Medication Distribution and Inventory Control Systems

Learning Outcomes

After completing this chapter, the technician should be able to:

- Describe distribution processes used in the inpatient and outpatient setting.
- Explain the role of the formulary in purchasing and inventory systems.
- Apply the proper principles and processes when receiving and storing pharmaceuticals.
- Identify key techniques for reviewing packaging, labeling, and storage conditions when handling pharmaceuticals.
- Describe the methods of inventory control that may be used to maintain adequate stocks of pharmaceuticals and medical devices.
- Demonstrate both an understanding of pharmaceutical products that require special handling within the purchasing and inventory system.
- Explain the ordering, receiving, and stocking process for pharmaceuticals and medical devices.
- Describe inventory procedures for recalled products, controlled substances, chemotherapy products, investigational drugs, and other products requiring special handling.
- Demonstrate an understanding of the appropriate processes in the handling of pharmaceutical recalls and the disposal of pharmaceutical products.
- Describe the characteristics of durable and nondurable medical equipment.

This chapter applies to Section II of the PTCB exam, Maintaining Medication and Inventory Control Systems.

The Formulary System

Most hospitals and health care systems develop a list of medications that may be prescribed for their patients. This list, usually called a *formulary*, serves as the cornerstone of the purchasing and inventory control system. The formulary is developed and maintained by a committee of medical and allied health staff called the Pharmacy and Therapeutics (P&T) Committee. This group generally consists of physicians, pharmacists, nurses, and administrators, although other disciplines may be present, including dieticians, risk managers, and case managers. The group collaborates to ensure that the safest, most efficacious, and least costly medications are included on the formulary. The products on the hospital formulary dictate what the hospital pharmacy should keep in inventory. Third-party prescription drug benefit providers (PBMs) will also establish plan-specific formularies for their ambulatory patients. Ambulatory (retail) pharmacy staff frequently encounter insurance plan–specific drug formularies in serving their customers and adjust their inventory accordingly. Most retail pharmacies do not restrict items in their inventory rigidly. This is because in this setting, inventories are largely dependent on the dynamic needs of their patient population and, to some degree, the patients' insurance plans. Therefore, the concept of formulary management differs greatly depending on the perspective (ie, that of the hospital compared with that of the retail pharmacy).

Nonformulary Protocol

Typically, when a prescriber orders a nonformulary product, the pharmacist requests verbal or written justification for its use and challenges the request, as appropriate, if a comparable or therapeutically equivalent product is available on the hospital formulary. In certain cases, the utilization of a nonformulary product is warranted when it is believed its benefit is superior to the other alternative formulary items that may exist (usually for a patient-specific or disease-specific reason). The P&T committee regularly reviews nonformulary drug utilization to identify trends and review concerns, and this process may prompt the addition of new products to the formulary over time.

Ordering Pharmaceuticals

Some pharmacies employ a dedicated purchasing agent to manage the procurement and inventory of pharmaceuticals. Others employ a more general approach whereby a variety of staff are involved in ordering pharmaceuticals. The state-of-the-art practice involves the use of computer and Internet technology to manage the process of purchasing and receiving pharmaceuticals from a drug wholesaler. This process includes online procurement and purchase order generation and electronic receiving processes that involve bar code technology and hand-held computer devices (Figure 2-1). Use of computer technology for these purposes has many benefits, including up-to-the-minute product availability information, comprehensive reporting capabilities, accuracy, and efficiency. Use of computer technology also facilitates compliance with various pharmaceutical purchasing contracts.

Receiving and Storing Pharmaceuticals

One of the most useful experiences for a new pharmacy technician is to witness the receipt of pharmaceuticals by the pharmacy department. This experience is useful for a number of reasons:

- It helps the pharmacy technician become familiar with various processes involved with the ordering and receipt of pharmaceuticals.
- It may help the technician become familiar with formulary items.
- It may demonstrate the system used to ensure that only formulary items are put into inventory.
- It helps familiarize the technician with the locations in which drugs are stored.

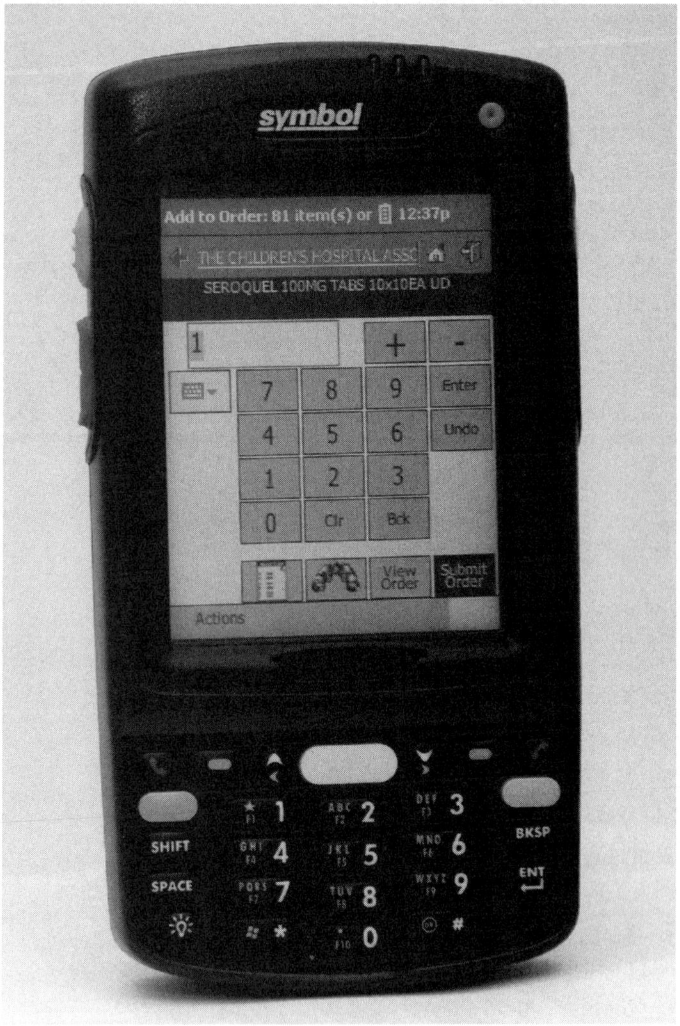

Figure 2-1. Handheld Bar Code Scanning Device.

Receiving is one of the most important parts of the pharmacy operation. A poorly organized and executed receiving system can put patients at risk and elevate health care costs. For example, if the wrong concentration of a product were received in error, it could lead to a dosing error or a delay in therapy. Misplaced products or out-of-stock products jeopardize patient care as well as the efficiency of the pharmacy—both undesirable and costly outcomes. To avoid these unfavorable outcomes, pharmacy technicians should become familiar with the process for receiving and storing pharmaceuticals.

The Receiving Process

Some pharmacies create processes whereby, as much as is possible, the person receiving pharmaceuticals is different from the individual ordering them. This is especially important for controlled substances because it effectively establishes a check in the system to minimize opportunities for drug diversion.

In a reliable and efficient receiving system, the receiving personnel verify that the shipment is complete and intact (ie, check for missing or damaged items) before putting items into circulation or inventory. The receiving process begins with the verification of the boxes containing pharmaceuticals delivered by the shipper. The person receiving the shipment verifies that the name and address on the boxes is correct and that the number of boxes matches the shipping manifest. Many drug wholesalers use rigid plastic crates because they protect the contents of each shipment better than foam or cardboard boxes. Plastic crates are also environmentally friendly because they are returned to the wholesaler for cleaning and reuse. In any case, each box should be inspected for gross damage.

Products with a cold storage requirement (ie, refrigeration or freezing) should be processed first (see Table 2-1 for storage temperatures). The shipper is responsible for ensuring the cold storage environment is maintained during shipping and will generally package these items in a transportable foam cooler. The shipper will include frozen cold packs to keep products at the correct storage temperature during shipment.

Receiving personnel play a critical role in protecting the pharmacy from financial responsibility for products damaged in shipment, products not ordered, and products not received. If there is any obvious damage or other discrepancies with the shipment, such as a breech in the cold storage environment or an incorrect product, they should be noted on the shipping manifest, and if warranted, the appropriate part of the shipment should be refused. Ideally, gross shipment damage or incorrect box counts should be identified in the presence of the delivery person and should be documented when signing for the order. Other problems identified after delivery personnel have left, such as mispicks, product dating, or internally damaged goods must be resolved according to the vendor's policies. Most vendors have specific procedures to follow in reporting and resolving such problems.

The next step of the receiving process entails checking the newly delivered products against the receiving copy of the purchase order. This generally occurs after the delivery person has left. For the supplier a purchase order, created when the order is placed, is a complete list of the items that were ordered. Some pharmacies may still use a traditional paper purchase order. However, the state-of-the-art practice employs electronic, Web-based technology to place orders with respective wholesale distributors (Figure 2-2). In this case, the order is transmitted and received in an instant, and the wholesaler's inventory of particular products is available in near real-time. This technology allows for more efficient operations and effective communication between the pharmacy and wholesaler, and simplifies order reconciliation and billing processes.

The person responsible for checking products into inventory uses the receiving copy to ensure that the products ordered have been received. The name, brand, dosage form, size of the package, concentration strength, and quantity of

Table 2-1. Defined Storage Temperatures and Humidity†

Freezer	−25° to −10° C	−13° to 14° F
Cold (Refrigerated)	2° to 8° C	36° to 46° F
Cool	8° to 15° C	46° to 59° F
Room Temperature	The temperature prevailing in a working area.	
Controlled Room Temperature	20° to 25° C	68° to 77° F
Warm	30° to 40° C	86° to 104° F
Excessive Heat	Any temperature above 40°C (104° F)	
Dry Place	A place that does not exceed 40 percent average relative humidity at controlled room temperature or the equivalent water vapor pressure at other temperatures. Storage in a container validated to protect the article from moisture vapor, including storage in bulk, is considered a dry place.	

† United States Pharmacopeia 26/The National Formulary 21, pp. 9–10; 2003. United States Pharmacopeial Convention, Inc., Rockville, MD.

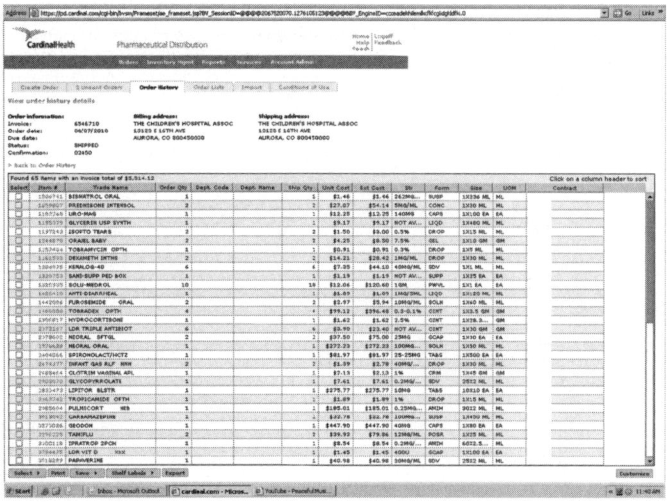

Figure 2-2. Electronic Purchase Order.

product must match the purchase order. Generally, once the accuracy of the shipment is confirmed, the purchase order copy is signed and dated by the person receiving the shipment. At this point, the product's expiration date should be checked to ensure that it meets the pharmacy's minimum expiration date requirement. Frequently, pharmacies will require that products received have a minimum 6 months' shelf life remaining before they expire. If a pharmacy uses a Barcode Medication Administration (BCMA) system, it is critical that each bar code is scanned at the time each product is received. This ensures the product bar code is in the BCMA system so it will scan correctly when it gets to the bedside. This applies even if the product has been received before from the same manufacturer. Some bar codes contain lot and expiration dating information, which could change with each manufacturer batch production. In the event a bar code does not scan, it is customary for the receiving technician to manually add the item to the BCMA system or overlay an internal bar code on the product prior to shelving it. It is noteworthy to mention that on occasion, the manufacturer/wholesaler may inadvertently ship an excess quantity of an ordered product to the pharmacy. The ethical response is to notify the manufacturer or wholesaler of this situation immediately and arrange for

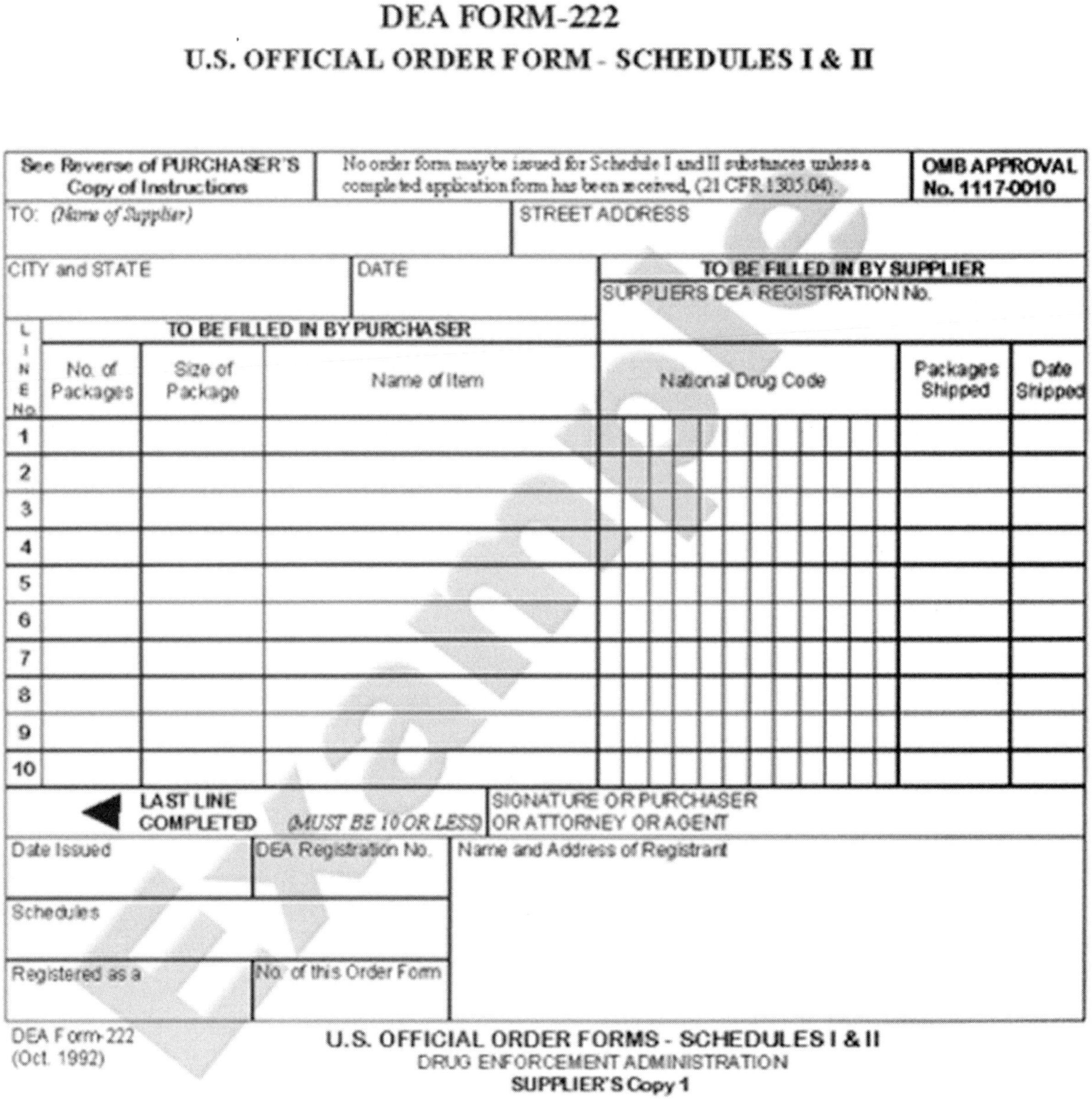
DEA FORM-222
U.S. OFFICIAL ORDER FORM - SCHEDULES I & II

See Reverse of PURCHASER'S Copy of Instructions
No order form may be issued for Schedule I and II substances unless a completed application form has been received, (21 CFR 1305.04).
OMB APPROVAL No. 1117-0010
TO: (Name of Supplier)
STREET ADDRESS
CITY and STATE
DATE
TO BE FILLED IN BY SUPPLIER
SUPPLIERS DEA REGISTRATION No.
TO BE FILLED IN BY PURCHASER

LINE No.	No. of Packages	Size of Package	Name of Item	National Drug Code	Packages Shipped	Date Shipped
1						
2						
3						
4						
5						
6						
7						
8						
9						
10						

LAST LINE COMPLETED (MUST BE 10 OR LESS)
SIGNATURE OR PURCHASER OR ATTORNEY OR AGENT
Date Issued
DEA Registration No.
Name and Address of Registrant
Schedules
Registered as a
No. of this Order Form
DEA Form-222 (Oct. 1992)
U.S. OFFICIAL ORDER FORMS - SCHEDULES I & II
DRUG ENFORCEMENT ADMINISTRATION
SUPPLIER'S Copy 1

Figure 2–3. DEA Form 222.

Received to stock
4 × 50's Oral Polio Vaccine, 0.5 ml
50 × 4's Haemophilus B vaccine vials
13 each Piperacillin 40 gm vials
30 DTP vials, 7.5 ml
4/15/97
One vial Piperacillin broken in shipment.
Joe Johnson
Pharmacy Technician

Receipt on blank piece of paper must include precise detail of the amount, product description, person receiving product, and the date of receipt.

Figure 2-4. Receipt of Pharmaceutical on Blank Paper.

the return of any excess quantity. Controlled substances require additional processing upon receipt. Regulations specific to Schedule II controlled substances require the completion of DEA form 222 (Figure 2-3) upon receipt of these products. The form must be filed separately with a copy of the invoice and packing slip accompanying each shipment. If a pharmacist or pharmacy technician other than the receiving technician removes a product from a shipment before it has been properly received and cannot locate the receiving copy of the purchase order, then a written record of receipt should be created. This is done by listing the product, dosage form, concentration or strength, package size, and quantity on a blank piece of paper (Figure 2-4) or on the supplier's packing slip or invoice and checking off the line item received (Figure 2-5). In both cases, the name of the person receiving the product should be included and the document should be given to the receiving technician to avoid confusion and an unnecessary call to the wholesaler or manufacturer.

Invoice

Shipper
Pharmaceutical Labs
185 Commerce Avenue
Ft. Washington, PA

Buyer
Community Hospital
1 Valley Road
Suburbia, MD 20777

Invoice # 12346
Invoice Date 4/01/97

Quantity		*Product #*	*Product Description*	*Unit Price*	*Amount*
5	4 rec.	6190	Orimune 50 × 1	$450.00	$2,250.00
4	✓	7183	Haemophilus B Vaccine	$ 52.92	$2,646.00
13	12 rec.	4391	Piperacillin 40 g Vial	$110.00	$1,320.00
30	✓	2727	DPT Vaccine 7.5ml Vial	$ 56.50	$1,695.00

Quantity received as indicated
one vial Piperacillin broken in shipment.
Received 4 × 50's Orimune
50 Haemophilus B Vaccine
13 Piperacillin 40 gm vial
30 DTP Vaccine 7.5 ml
4/15/97
Joe Johnson
Pharmacy Technician

Receipt on an invoice or packing slip can be done the same way as receipt on a blank piece of paper or the quantities can be checked or modified as received.

Figure 2-5. Receipt of Pharmaceutical on Packing Slip/Invoice.

The Storing Process

Once the product has been properly received, it must be properly stored. Depending on the size and type of the pharmacy operation, the product may be placed in a bulk central storage area or in the active dispensing areas of the pharmacy. In any case, the expiration date of the product should be compared with the products currently in stock. Products in stock that have expired should be removed. Products that will expire in the near future should be highlighted and placed in the front of the shelf or bin. This is a common practice known as *stock rotation*. The newly acquired products will generally have longer shelf lives and should be placed behind products that will expire before them. Stock rotation is an important inventory management principle that promotes the use of products before they expire and helps prevent the use of expired products and waste.

Product Handling Considerations

Pharmacy technicians usually spend more time handling and preparing medications than do pharmacists. This situation presents pharmacy technicians with the critical responsibility of assessing and evaluating each product from both a content and labeling standpoint. It also gives technicians an opportunity to confirm that the receiving process was performed properly.

Just as checking the product label carefully at the time a prescription or medication order is filled is important, so is taking the same care when receiving and storing pharmaceuticals. It is best to read product packaging carefully rather than rely on the general appearance of the product (eg, packaging type, size or shape, color, logo), because a product's appearance may change frequently and may be similar to other products. Technicians play a vital role in minimizing dispensing errors caused by human fallibility. Technicians are generally the first in a series of double checks involved in an accurate dispensing process.

When performing purchasing or inventory management roles, the technician must pay close attention to the product's expiration date. For liquids or injectable products, color and clarity should also be checked for consistency with the product standard. Products with visible particles, an unusual appearance, or a broken seal should be reported to the pharmacist.

Because pharmacy technicians handle so many products each day, they are in a perfect position to identify packaging and storage issues that could lead to errors. Technicians must pay close attention to three main issues:

- *Similar drug names*—Various drugs with similar names can cause problems when stored in an immediately adjacent shelf position. All staff members should be alerted to look-alike or sound-alike products.
- *Similar package sizes*—Stocking products of similar name, color, shape, and size can result in error if someone fails to read the label correctly. Sometimes the company name or log is emphasized on the label instead of the drug name, concentration, or strength.
- *Similar label format*—Storing products that are similar in appearance adjacent to one another can result in error if someone fails to read the label.

Alerting other staff members to products that fall into one of these categories is essential. Some pharmacies routinely discuss product-handling considerations at staff meetings or in departmental newsletters. Dispensing errors may be averted by simply relocating a look-alike/sound-alike product to a different shelf location or placing warning notes (ie, auxiliary labeling or highlights) on the shelf or on the product itself. Pharmacy technicians should also discuss their concerns with coworkers and may advocate changes to products with poor labeling with the manufacturer.

Maintaining and Managing Inventory

An inventory management system is an organized approach designed to maintain just the right amount of pharmaceutical products in the pharmacy at all times. A variety of inventory management systems are used, ranging from simple to complex. They include employing an order book where pharmacy staff simply write down what they believe is necessary to order (aka the "eyeball" method), the minimum/maximum (par) level, the Pareto (ABC) Analysis, and the fully automated, computerized system.

Economic Models

The Pareto ABC system, also known as the *80/20 rule*, relies on the premise that managing 20% of the inventory will cover 80% of the costs (Figure 2-6). It essentially groups inventory products by aggregate value and volume of use into three groupings (A, B, and C). This analysis is useful to determine where inventory control efforts are best directed. For example, Group A may include 20% of all items that make up 65% of the inventory cost. Tight control over these items would be sensible. Group B may include 30% of items that make up 25% of the inventory cost. An automatic order cycle here based on well-established par levels might be useful. Group C may include 50% of items that make up 10% of the inventory cost. Less aggressive monitoring of these items may be justifiable.

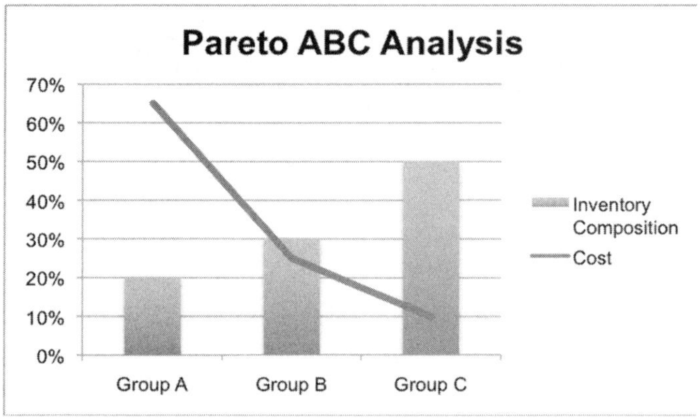

Figure 2-6. Pareto ABC Analysis.

Manual Systems

Manual inventory models require the active oversight of pharmacy technicians and are usually based on a minimum/maximum, or par-level, system. The **par-level system** uses predetermined stock minimum and maximum quantities to be maintained. Once item par-levels are established, they are usually identified on or near the shelf label of individual pharmaceutical items kept in inventory (Figure 2-7). Staff members can create a pharmaceutical order using a hand-held bar code scanning device or enter product stock numbers directly into a personal computer. They strive to maintain physical pharmaceutical inventories within the minimum to maximum range to avoid running short on a product or overstocking. Running short on a product can affect patient care, and overstocking adds unnecessary operational expense.

Manual systems require pharmacy staff to routinely scan inventory levels and place orders accordingly. With both electronic and manual systems, pharmacy staff should be aware that the diversity of their patients' specific needs or dynamic seasonal volume may require modification in a particular product's par-level.

Automation

In contrast to a manual system, with an automated perpetual inventory system, each dispensing transaction is subtracted from the perpetual inventory that is maintained

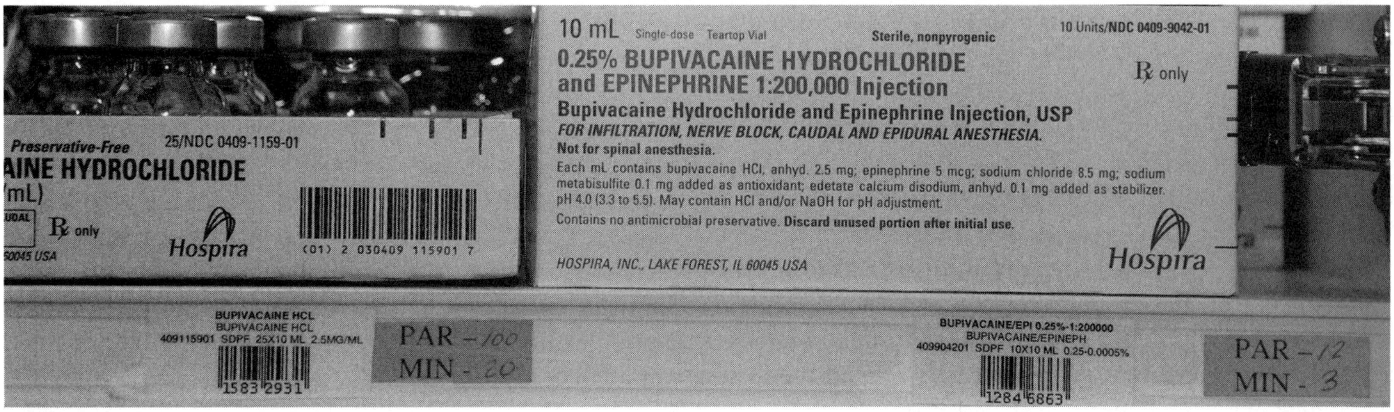

Figure 2-7. Shelf labels correspond to each product and are placed on the storage bin or shelf. The minimum and maximum inventory level is written on this label, and the information is used as a relative guide for pharmacy staff involved in purchasing pharmaceuticals.

electronically in a computerized database; conversely, quantities of products received are automatically added to the inventory on hand in the computerized system. When the quantity of a pharmaceutical product in stock reaches a predetermined point (often called par) a purchase order is automatically generated to order more of the product. The system does not depend on any one employee to monitor the inventory or reorder pharmaceuticals.

The technology is available to have a computerized inventory in most pharmacies, but interfacing a computerized inventory system with existing pharmacy computer systems designed for dispensing and patient management systems is often difficult. In addition, other variables, such as product availability, contract changes, and changing use patterns (either up or down), make relying on the fully computerized model challenging. Consequently, even the most sophisticated electronic and automated systems still require human oversight.

Automated dispensing devices are capable of tracking perpetual inventory at the product level. They also limit access to only authorized personnel and record the identities of individuals who access inventory, as well as how much of a specific drug was removed for a given patient. A useful feature in many of these systems allows pharmacy personnel to automatically generate a fill-list of what needs to be replenished on the basis of a par-level system. The par-level inventory system relies on a predetermined order quantity and an order point. These systems typically include shelf labels that correspond to each product and are placed on the storage bin or shelf to alert staff to the minimum stock quantity (see Figure 2-7). The minimum and maximum inventory level is written on this label, and the information is used as a relative guide for pharmacy staff involved in purchasing.

The use of automated dispensing devices in inpatient hospital nursing units, clinics, operating rooms, and emergency rooms has facilitated the use of computers for inventory management. Similar devices are evolving for the retail pharmacy and hold promise for making the dispensing process safer and more efficient, and also assisting in inventory management. These devices are essentially repositories, or *pharmaceutical vending machines,* for medications that will be dispensed directly from a patient care area. A variety of manufacturers of automated dispensing devices are in the market today—the Pyxis Medstation®, Meditrol®, Omnicell®, MED Carousel (Figure 2-8), and SureMed® are some examples.

These machines are generally networked via a dedicated computer file server within the facility. They allow both unit-dose and bulk pharmaceuticals to be stocked

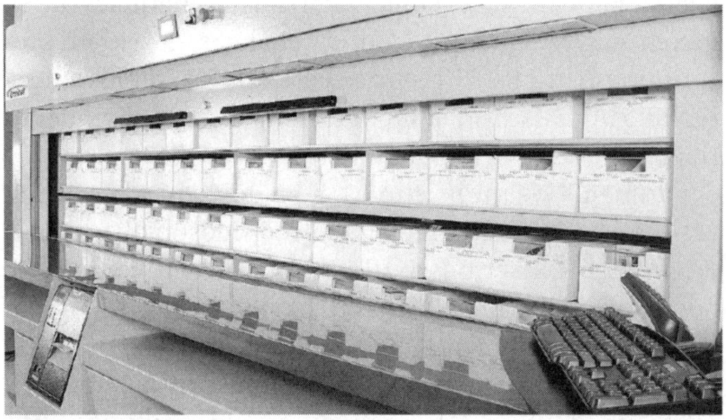

Figure 2-8. Medication dispensing carousel.

securely on a given patient care unit location. Each unit's inventory is configurable and allows for variation and flexibility from device to device depending on its location. The machines are capable of tracking perpetual inventory at the product level. They also limit access to authorized personnel, record the identities of those who access inventory, and record how much was removed for each patient. A useful feature in many of these systems allows pharmacy personnel to generate automatically a fill-list of what needs to be replenished based on a par-level system. In essence, the nursing and medical personnel who use these automated dispensing devices have a computerized inventory and billing system that the pharmacy staff manages. Medications used to restock these devices may be taken from the pharmacy's main inventory, or a separate purchase order may be executed periodically for each device.

Just-in-time inventory management is a philosophy that simply means products are ordered and delivered at just the right time—when they are needed for patient care—with a goal of minimizing wasted steps, labor, and cost. Pharmaceuticals are neither overstocked nor understocked. In pharmacy, this business philosophy couples responsible financial management of pharmaceutical purchasing with the clinical aspects of patient care.

Many pharmacies use an order book system, also called a *want list* or *want book.* When pharmacists or pharmacy technicians determine that a product should be reordered, they write the item in the order book. Although this approach is simple, it also provides the least amount of organized control over inventory. Its success is highly dependent on the participation of staff. Therefore, it is usually not the sole method of inventory management and is often used in conjunction with one of the other systems mentioned.

Regardless of the inventory system used, pharmacy technicians are vital contributors. The pharmacy technician may frequently identify changes in use or prescription patterns of pharmaceuticals. Examples might include high use of asthmatic medications (ie, epinephrine, albuterol, or inhaled steroids) by the emergency department or various clinics, high doses of a particular antibiotic (eg, chloramphenicol or liposomal amphotericin b) for a seriously ill patient who is likely to be hospitalized for an extended period, or high-dose opioid use by one or more oncology patients. Alerting purchasing staff to orders for unusual amounts of medications helps avoid out-of-stock situations and facilitates optimal inventory management.

Drug Recalls

A drug recall effectively removes a manufactured product from the market.

Manufacturers, on their own accord or at the direction of the Food and Drug Administration (FDA), occasionally *recall* pharmaceuticals for such reasons as mislabeling, contamination, lack of potency, lack of adherence to the acceptable good manufacturing practices, or other situations that may present a significant risk to public health. A pharmacy must have a system for rapid removal of any recalled products.

Role of the FDA

The FDA plays an active role in initiating the drug-recall process. Unlike biologics and devices, the FDA has no statutory (legal) authority to recall drugs. Manufacturers voluntarily issue recalls in their duty to protect public health and the FDA helps manufacturers coordinate drug recall information and develop specific voluntary recall plans. It performs health hazard evaluations to assess public risk associated with products being recalled (Table 2-2).

Role of Pharmacy, Manufacturers, and Distributors

Because of their responsibility to protect the public consumer, manufacturers and distributors typically implement voluntary recalls when a marketed drug product needs to be removed from the market. Recall notices are sent in writing to pharmacies by the manufacturer of the product or by drug wholesalers. These notices indicate the class of recall, the reason for recall, the name of the recalled product, the manufacturer, all affected lot numbers of the product, response required, instructions on the extent of action required in contacting affected patients, and how to return the product to the manufacturer.

On receipt of the recall notice, a pharmacy staff member, usually a pharmacy technician, checks all pharmaceutical inventory stores to determine if any recalled products

Table 2-2. FDA Drug Recall Classes

FDA Drug Recall Classes	
Class I	The most serious of recalls; ongoing product use may result in serious health threat or death.
Class II	Moderate severity concern; ongoing product use may pose serious adverse events or irreversible consequences.
Class III	Lowest severity concern; ongoing product use unlikely to cause adverse health threat; however, a marginal chance of injury may exist, so the product is being recalled.

are in stock. If a recalled product is in stock, all products should be gathered, packaged, and returned to the manufacturer if requested. In some cases, the drug will simply be destroyed. The instructions and product package should be reviewed by the pharmacist-in-charge before returning it to the manufacturer or distributor. If patients have received a recalled product, the pharmacist-in-charge has a duty to follow the action required by the recall notice. Upon completion of all activity regarding the product recall, a summary of actions taken should be documented on the recall letter and filed in the pharmaceutical recall log. The FDA has been known to request documentation of all recall activities to ensure compliance, and ultimately patient safety. The technician should keep in mind that it may be necessary to order replacement stock to compensate for recalled items that were removed from stock.

Drug Shortages

Often, manufacturers will be unable to supply a pharmaceutical because of various supply and demand situations. These situations may involve the inability to obtain raw materials, manufacturing difficulties related to equipment failure, or simply an inability to produce sufficient quantities to stay ahead of market demand. Although unfortunate, it is a reality that must be dealt with to avoid compromising patient care. As with drug recalls, the pharmacist in charge should be notified so he or she may communicate drug shortages and recommend alternative therapies to prescribers.

Counterfeit Pharmaceuticals

Unfortunately, there is a global concern related to the fraudulent mislabeling and distribution of counterfeit drugs. These products are dangerous because they may not meet standards of quality or potency and are therefore harmful or ineffective in treating the disease for which they are intended. These products can range from those containing incorrect ingredients, sub-potency, and even toxic ingredients, even though the package or dosage form appears to be legitimate. Obviously, these products are illegal and pose serious threats to the patient and caregiver. Any pharmaceutical product is at risk for being counterfeited, and developing countries appear to be the most threatened by this malicious activity. Unfortunately, the level of sophistication of individuals engaged in the act of counterfeiting is growing, even in countries with more highly controlled markets, including the United States. In 2006, the World Health Organization formed an initiative aimed at combating counterfeit medication distribution. It is a global partnership called *International Medicinal Products Anti-Counterfeiting Taskforce* (IMPACT). The organization has brought together international enforcement and regulatory agencies, customs and police authorities, pharmaceutical manufacturing representatives, wholesale companies, health-care providers, and patient delegates to coordinate efforts and raise awareness of this problem. As a result, laws, standards, monitoring and reporting programs, and penal sanctions are being developed and coordinated to minimize the threat of fraudulent medication distribution. In many states, pedigree laws have either been passed or are in the pipeline. Simply stated, these laws require the drug wholesaler to provide a statement of origin or otherwise prove the genealogy of drugs distributed. Every step in the distribution chain will have to be documented and verified, from the point of manufacturer origin all the way to the wholesale distribution point. An electronic pedigree (e-Pedigree) ensures through documentation that a drug was safely and securely manufactured and distributed.

Pharmacy technicians need to be aware of the existence of counterfeit pharmaceuticals and the methods that are being employed to address the issue. When managing drug shortages and working outside of the routine wholesale distribution channels, it is essential to ensure that pharmaceuticals are being obtained from a reliable source. It is acceptable to obtain and verify the licensing information from alternative drug suppliers, or those purporting to have product when other, reputable suppliers do not. The technician should also remain aware of those pharmaceutical products known or suspected to be at risk and communicate any concerns when procuring, receiving, and handling these products.

? Pop Quiz!

A prescription indicates 1 tab q 3–4 h prn pain, dispense #30. What is the EDS?

Ordering and Borrowing Pharmaceuticals

Pharmaceutical Purchasing (Buying) Groups

Most health-system pharmacies are members of a group purchasing organization (GPO). Health systems and hospitals join together in a purchasing group to leverage their buying power and take advantage of lower prices manufacturers offer to large groups that can guarantee a significant volume of orders over long periods of time (typically 1 to 2 years). Retail chain pharmacies are also able to negotiate better pricing on the basis of volume. Contracts may involve sole-source or multisource products. Sole-source products are products available from only one manufacturer, whereas multisource products (frequently termed *generic* products) are available from numerous manufacturers. Sole-source products may be produced by only one manufacturer; however, they may be included in what is known as a *competitive market basket* (eg, proton-pump-inhibitors, such as omeprazole and lansoprazole) when there are competing brand-name products on the market.

GPOs negotiate purchasing contracts that are mutually favorable to members of the group and to manufacturers. In addition to lower prices, pharmacies benefit from reduced time staff spent establishing and managing purchasing contracts with product vendors. A GPO guarantees the price for pharmaceuticals over the established contract period, which may be 1 or more years. With the purchase price predetermined, the pharmacy can order the product directly from the manufacturer or from a wholesale supplier. Occasionally, manufacturers are unable to supply a given product that the pharmacy is buying on contract. The pharmacy may then have to buy or substitute a competing product not on contract at a higher cost. Most purchasing contracts will include language to protect the pharmacy from incurring additional expenses in this event. Generally, the manufacturer will be liable to rebate the difference in cost back to the pharmacy. Therefore, it is important for the pharmacy technician to document any off-contract purchases and share them with the pharmacist-in-charge for reconciliation with the contracted vendor.

Direct Purchasing

Direct purchasing from a manufacturer involves the execution of a purchase order (P.O.) between the pharmacy and the manufacturer. The advantages of direct purchasing include not having to pay handling fees to a third-party wholesaler, the ability to order on an infrequent basis (eg, once a month), and a less demanding system for monitoring inventory. Some disadvantages include the need for a large storage capacity; a large amount of cash invested in inventory; the complication of the pharmacy's return/credit process; and staff resources required in the pharmacy and accounts payable department to prepare, process, and pay purchase orders to more companies. Other disadvantages have to do with the likelihood that the manufacturer's warehouse is not located near the pharmacy. The manufacturers depend on shipping firms to ship products reliably; however, delivery is often unpredictable or not available on weekends, and there may be delays in delivery.

For most pharmacies, the disadvantages of direct ordering outweigh the advantages. As a result, most pharmacies primarily purchase through a drug wholesaler. There are, however, some drugs that can only be purchased directly from the manufacturers. These products generally require unique control or storage conditions. Consequently, most pharmacies will have a combination of direct purchases from manufacturers and purchases from drug wholesalers.

Drug Wholesaler Purchasing/Prime Vendor Purchasing

Purchasing from a drug wholesaler permits the acquisition of drug products from different manufacturers through a single vendor. When a health-system pharmacy agrees to purchase the majority (90 to 95%) of its pharmaceuticals from a single wholesale company, a prime vendor arrangement is established, and, customarily, a contract between the pharmacy and the drug wholesaler is developed. Usually, the wholesaler agrees to deliver at least 95 to 98% of the items on schedule and offers 24-hour/7-day-per-week emergency service. The wholesaler also provides the pharmacy with electronic order entry or receiving devices, a computer system for ordering, barcoded shelf stickers, and a printer for order confirmation printouts. It may also offer a highly competitive discount (minus 1 to 2%) below product cost and contract pricing and competitive alternate contract pricing. Some wholesalers will offer even larger discounts to pharmacies that may prefer a prepayment arrangement. In these situations, the wholesaler monitors the aggregate purchases of the pharmacy (eg, a rolling 3-month average) and bills the pharmacy this amount in advance (prepayment). This arrangement creates larger cash flow and investment capital for the wholesaler while saving the pharmacy money on its pharmaceutical purchases.

These wholesaler services make the establishment of a prime vendor contract appealing and result in the following advantages: more timely ordering and delivery, less time spent creating purchase orders, fewer inventory carrying costs, less documentation, computer-generated lists of pharmaceuticals purchased, and overall simplification of the credit and return process. Purchasing through a prime vendor customarily allows for drugs to be received shortly before use, supporting the just-in-time ordering philosophy mentioned earlier in this chapter. Purchasing from a wholesaler is thus a highly efficient and cost-effective approach toward pharmaceutical purchasing and inventory management.

Borrowing Pharmaceuticals

No matter how effective a purchasing system is, the pharmacy occasionally must borrow drugs from other pharmacies. Most pharmacies have policies and procedures addressing this situation. Borrowing or loaning drugs between pharmacies is usually restricted to emergency situations and limited to authorized staff. Borrowing is also limited to products that are commercially available, thus eliminating such items as compounded products or investigational medications. Most pharmacies have developed forms to document and track merchandise that is borrowed or loaned. These forms also help staff document the details necessary for error-free transactions.

The pharmacy's borrow and loan policies and procedures should provide detailed directions on how to borrow and loan products, which products may be borrowed or loaned, sources for them, and reconciliation of borrow-loan transactions (the payback process). Securing the borrowed item may require the use of a transport or courier service or may include the use of security staff or other designated personnel. This information is vital for pharmacy technicians to understand so they can fulfill their responsibility when borrowing and loaning products.

Pop Quiz!

What form is required to order OxyContin tablets?

Products Requiring Special Handling

Most pharmaceuticals, with the exception of controlled substances, investigational drugs, compounded products, repackaged drugs, and drug samples will be handled and processed in the inventorying and purchasing systems described above.

Controlled Substances

Controlled substances have specific ordering, receiving, storage, dispensing, inventory, record-keeping, return, waste, and disposal requirements established under the law. The *Pharmacist's Manual: An Informational Outline of the Controlled Substances Act of 1970* and the *ASHP Technical Assistance Bulletin on Institutional Use of Controlled Substances* provide detailed information on the specific handling requirements for controlled substances.

The pharmacy technician should know two principles regarding controlled substances:

1. Ordering and receiving Schedule II controlled substances requires special order forms and additional time (1 to 3 days).
2. These substances are inventoried and tracked continuously. This type of inventory method is referred to as a perpetual inventory process, whereby each dose or packaged unit, such as a tablet, vial, or ml of fluid volume is accounted for at all times.

In some pharmacies, pharmacy technicians work with pharmacists to manage inventory and order, dispense, store, and control narcotics and other controlled substances. Controlled substances require additional processing when ordering, receiving, dispensing, storing, and inventorying occurs. These procedures are required by Drug Enforcement Administration (DEA) regulations, and in many cases, the state board of pharmacy. These regulations create the chain of accountability in the interest of minimizing drug diversion, illicit drug use, and public safety. State and federal regulations vary regarding length of storage requirements for purchase orders, invoices, and dispensing records. It is best to check both sets of regulations and comply with the stricter requirements.

Regulations specific to Schedule II controlled substances require DEA form 222 to be completed to initiate procurement of these products. Form 222 is a triplicate, hand-written form and each copy has a specific intent, as specified by the DEA. On receipt of DEA Schedule II products, the pharmacy must separately file the appropriate copy of the form 222, along with the supplier's copy of the invoice and packing slip accompanying each shipment. Alternatively, the pharmacy can be registered with the DEA to place Schedule II orders online through the wholesaler's electronic process. Schedule III, IV, and V controlled substances are generally obtained in a manner identical to other noncontrolled substances. However, the receipt and storage requirements of these products may depend on state regulation or the specific employer's policy. For example, state regulation may require a pharmacy to file separately the receipts of all controlled substances ordered during a particular year and maintain them in a readily retrievable manner for inspection. Some pharmacies may require all controlled substance inventories to be shelved separately from other legend drugs, whereas others may store them together.

Chemotherapy

Because of the hazards inherent with human exposure to antineoplastic or chemotherapy products, care and precaution must be exercised in the receipt, handling, and storage of these products. The distributor will generally ship antineoplastic drugs separate and apart from other products (eg, in their own container). Special care should be exercised when opening and unpacking totes containing these products. Although the distributor will take appropriate measures to properly pack and pad the items inside totes, it is still possible for damage to occur. Pharmacy technicians should be familiar with the organization's chemotherapy and hazardous materials spill management protocol. Most hospitals will have a "chemotherapy spill kit" on hand to be used in the management and cleanup of an accidental spill.

Investigational Drugs

Investigational drugs also require special ordering, inventorying, and handling procedures. Generally, the use of investigational drugs is categorized into two distinct areas:

1. Investigational drugs used in a formal protocol that was approved by the institution
2. Investigational drugs used for a single patient on a one-time basis that have been authorized by the manufacturer and the FDA

In both cases, the physician may be responsible for the ordering and the pharmacy staff handles the inventory management of the investigational drug. Some pharmacies associated with academic affiliations or institutions conducting clinical research may have formally organized Investigational Drug Services managed by a pharmacist principally dedicated to pharmaceutical research activities. In these cases, the investigational drug service pharmacist may be responsible for the ordering, dispensing, and inventory management of investigational drugs according to the research protocol. Pharmacy technicians often prepare or handle investigational drugs and participate in the required perpetual inventory record-keeping system. Again, it is important for pharmacy technicians to learn the department procedures for investigational drugs and to be competent in the handling, storage, dispensing, and inventory systems involved.

Restricted Drug Distribution System (RDDS)

The intent of the restricted drug distribution system is to ensure that specific drugs identified as high risk are safely procured, prescribed, dispensed, and administered. The FDA, the manufacturer, and the distributor collaborate to establish tighter controls over designated products.

If improperly administered, certain drugs can cause serious adverse effects, such as blood disorders, birth defects, or changes in cardiovascular status. Satisfying the requirements necessary to obtain these drugs may be limited to the presence of a specific disease state being treated by a physician who is registered under the RDDS. As a matter of satisfying restricted distribution requirements, the physician may have to attest to patient-specific criteria. This might include a failed treatment response to other medications, contraindications to other therapy, or provided laboratory data. In other cases, the physician may need to commit to administering the medication under controlled conditions, such as in their office.

In most cases, the RDDS will require:

- registration of the prescribing physician
- dispensing pharmacy
- patient name and other demographic information
- a patient agreement form for liability purposes
- the specific indication for the medication
- its dose and quantity to be dispensed

In some programs, lab results, adherence to a robust patient counseling or outreach protocol, and reimbursement information guaranteeing payment is required (Table 2-3). The primary goal of RDDS is safe, effective product use and reduced risk to the patient.

Compounded Products

Compounded pharmaceuticals are another type of product handled by pharmacy personnel. Unlike drugs ordered from an outside source, compounded products are extemporaneously prepared in the pharmacy as indicated by scientific compounding formulas. These products may include oral liquids, topical preparations, solid dosage forms, and sterile products.

Table 2–3. Examples of Restricted Distribution Products

	Specific Requirements					
Drug	Physician Enrollment and Training	Patient Enrollment	Requires Registration of Retail Pharmacy to Dispense	Specialty Distributor or Centralized Pharmacy	Administration in Medical Setting	Requires Lab Test Prior to Distribution
Abarelix (Plenaxis)	X		X*		X+	
Alosetron (Lotronex)	X					
Ambrisentan (Letairis)	X	X	X			X^^
Bosentan (Tracleer)	X	X		X		
Clozapine (Clozaril)	X	X	X			X^
Deferasirox (Exjade)	X			X		
Dofetilide (Tikosyn)	X	X	X		X++	
Getfitinib (Iressa)	X	X		X		
Isotretinoin (Accutane)	X	X	X			X^^
Lenalidomide (Revlimid)	X	X		X		X^^
Mifepristone (Mifeprex)	X				X+	
Nataluzimab (Tysabri)	X			X**		
Sodium Oxybate (Xyrem)	X	X		X		
Thalidomide (Thalomid)	X	X	X			X^^

* dispensed by registered hospital pharmacy
** dispensed only to authorized infusion sites
\+ administered in doctor's office
++ 3-day in-patient hospital stay required upon initiation
^ white blood cell count
^^ negative pregnancy test

The use of these products requires that prescribing patterns and expiration dates be monitored closely. Compounded products typically have short expiration dates, ranging from days to months. Because pharmacy technicians are likely to identify usage patterns and determine stock and product needs, procedures for monitoring patient use, product expiration dates, and additional stock needs must be well known and adhered to by technicians to prevent stock shortages. Specific pharmacy technicians may initiate compounding activities, but this may vary according to departmental procedures.

All chemicals are shipped according to Department of Transportation (DOT) and company safe practice standards, and include a materials safety data sheet (MSDS) for each chemical. Strong acids and alkaline chemicals and other toxic raw materials are frequently used in the process of compounding pharmaceuticals. The receiving pharmacy technician should be familiar with the utility and safe product handling and storage requirements of these chemicals.

Repackaged Pharmaceuticals

Although manufacturers supply many drugs in a prepackaged unit-dose form, the pharmacy staff is responsible for packaging some products. These items are generally unit-dose tablets and capsules, unit-dose oral liquids, and some bulk packages of oral solids and liquids. Each pharmacy establishes stocking mechanisms for these products and relies on pharmacy technicians to identify and respond to production and stock needs. Generally, designated technicians coordinate prepackaging activities, but some pharmacies may integrate repackaging with other pharmacy technician responsibilities. Knowledge of the pharmacy's procedures for repackaging is required to prevent disruptions in dispensing activities.

Nonformulary Items

Nonformulary items also require special handling. Nonformulary medications generally are not mixed into the shelving system of formulary products in the pharmacy; they fall outside normal inventorying mechanisms. Often, manual tracking mechanisms and computer system queries of active nonformulary orders are the two most common techniques used to monitor and order these products.

Medication Samples

The last products requiring special handling are medication samples. Traditional inventory management and handling practices do not work well with medication samples for two reasons:

1. Medication samples are not ordered by the pharmacy; the drug manufacturer usually provides them to physicians, upon request, free of charge. This often occurs without the pharmacy's knowledge.
2. Samples are not usually dispensed by the pharmacy.

These factors make it difficult to know whom to contact if a medication sample is recalled and to ensure that medication samples are not sold. Because of difficulties in controlling samples, organizations may allow samples to be stored and dispensed in ambulatory clinics only after the samples are registered with the pharmacy for tracking purposes. These difficult logistical and control factors have led many organizations to adopt policies that simply disallow medication samples altogether.

If your organization does allow medication samples, they will probably be stored outside the pharmacy, and pharmacy personnel will be required to register and inspect the stock. Pharmacy technicians are sometimes involved in inspecting medication sample storage units. These technicians are often responsible for determining if a sample is registered with the pharmacy, stored in acceptable quantities, labeled with an expiration date that has not been exceeded, and stored under acceptable conditions. Review your pharmacy's policies and procedures regarding medication samples to learn the role of the pharmacy technician. Many hospitals strive to maintain compliance with the standards of the Joint Commission on Accreditation of Healthcare Organizations (JCAHO). Its standards on *Medication Management* are intended to promote consistently safe practices related to the procurement, storage, dispensing, and administration of pharmaceuticals, and the use of sample drug products falls into this standard.

Radiopharmaceuticals

Radiopharmaceutical agents are typically used in diagnostic imaging as contrast media and can include oral and injectable products. Other radiopharmaceutical products are used therapeutically to treat diseases of the thyroid gland and forms of cancer. Technically speaking, these drugs are radioactive and potentially hazardous to humans and the environment, because they emit low to moderate levels of radiation. Therefore, special procedures aimed at minimizing exposure are warranted. Pharmacy technicians should become intimately familiar with and closely follow policies and procedures associated with the procurement, handling, and storage of radiopharmaceutical products. See *Manual for Pharmacy Technicians*, 4th ed., Chapter 6 ("Specialty Pharmacy Practice for additional information").

? Pop Quiz!

A patient brings in a prescription for Lantus U-100 insulin pens; dispense 1 box of 5 pens. The patient is to use 20 units Q AM. What is the EDS?

Proper Disposal and Return of Pharmaceuticals

Expired Pharmaceuticals

The most common reason drugs are returned to the manufacturer is because they have expired. The process for returning drugs in the original manufacturer packaging is relatively simple and not particularly time-consuming when done routinely. Returning expired products to the manufacturer or wholesaler prevents the inadvertent use of these products and enables the pharmacy to receive either full or partial credit for them. Some wholesalers limit credit given on returns of short-dated products. Generally, wholesalers will not give full credit on returns of products that will expire within 6 months. To return products, pharmacy personnel must complete the documentation required by the product's manufacturer or wholesaler and package the product for shipment. Many wholesalers have implemented electronic documentation systems to further simplify the return process. Technicians often perform these duties under the supervision of a pharmacist. Some pharmacies contract with an outside vendor that completes the documentation and coordinates the return of these products for a fee. In this case, the pharmacy technician need only assist the returned goods vendor with locating and packaging the expired pharmaceuticals. Many states are now enforcing regulations issued in the 1970s by the Environmental Protection Agency under the Resource Conservation and Recovery Act (RCRA) that govern the proper disposal mechanisms of hazardous chemicals, including drugs. Thus, each pharmacy should have detailed procedures governing the proper, legal disposal of pharmaceutical waste. The pharmacy technician should be familiar with these procedures. Disposal of expired compounded or repackaged pharmaceuticals by the pharmacy technician should be completed under the supervision of the pharmacist.

Pharmaceuticals compounded or repackaged by the pharmacy cannot be returned and must be disposed of after they have expired. It is important to dispose of these products for safety reasons. Proper disposal prevents the use of subpotent products or products whose sterility can no longer be guaranteed. The precise procedure for disposal depends on the type and content of the product. Some products, such as expired repackaged solids, can be disposed of via the general trash removal system, while others, such as expired compounded cytotoxic products, must be disposed of according to hazardous waste removal procedures. Each pharmacy has detailed procedures for hazardous waste removal, and the pharmacy technician should be familiar with these procedures. Disposal of expired compounded or repackaged pharmaceuticals by the pharmacy technician should be completed under the supervision of the pharmacist.

Other products requiring disposal rather than return are chemicals used in the pharmacy laboratory. Most pharmacies stock a supply of chemical-grade products used in extemporaneous pharmaceutical compounding. Examples of chemical products include sodium benzoate or sodium citrate (preservatives), lactose or talc (excipients), buffers, and active ingredients such as hydrocortisone, triamcinolone, neomycin, or lidocaine powders. When such products expire, they should be disposed of in accordance with the pharmacy's hazardous waste procedures.

Expired controlled substances are disposed of in a unique way. These products may not be returned to the manufacturer or wholesaler for credit. They must be destroyed, and the destruction must be documented to the satisfaction of the Drug Enforcement Administration (DEA). The DEA provides a form, titled "Registrant's Inventory of Drugs Surrendered" (Form 41, Figure 2-9) for recording the disposal of expired controlled substances. Ideally, the actual disposal of expired controlled substances should be completed by a company sanctioned by the DEA or by a representative of the state board of pharmacy. In other cases, the DEA may allow the destruction of controlled substances by a pharmacy, provided an appropriate witness process is followed and documented. The DEA form for disposal of controlled substances should be completed properly and submitted to the DEA immediately after the disposal has occurred. A DEA representative signs a copy of the record of disposal form and returns it to the pharmacy, where it is kept on file. Previously, the DEA allowed for shipment of expired controlled substances and the completed disposal form to the regional DEA office, but this practice is no longer permitted.

The use and disposition of investigational drugs must also be documented carefully. Expired investigational drugs should be returned to the manufacturer or sponsor of an investigational drug study according to the instructions they provide. The pharmacy technician may be responsible, under the supervision of the pharmacist, for documenting, packaging, and shipping the expired investigational agents. Investigational drug products that expire because of product instability or sterility issues should never be discarded. These doses should be retained with the investigational drug stock and be clearly marked as expired drug products, because the investigational study sponsor will need to review and account for all expired investigational drug products.

Pharmaceuticals that need to be returned because of an ordering error require authorization from the original supplier and the appropriate forms. The Prescription Drug Marketing Act mandates that pharmacies retain the authorization and retention records of returned pharmaceuticals in order to prevent diversion of pharmaceuticals. The pharmacy technician must be familiar with pharmacy procedures for returning medications to a supplier. Typically, a pharmacy will have a process for returning misordered medications to the prime drug wholesaler on a routine basis. This prevents the need to store overstocked or misordered products in the pharmacy. The pharmacy technician may be responsible for relevant documentation, filing of paperwork, and the packaging of returned products under the supervision of the pharmacist.

Pharmaceutical Waste Management

The environmental impact of pharmaceutical waste is becoming a prominent public health issue worldwide.

OMB Approval No. 1117 - 0007	U. S. Department of Justice / Drug Enforcement Administration **REGISTRANTS INVENTORY OF DRUGS SURRENDERED**	PACKAGE NO.

The following schedule is an inventory of controlled substances which is hereby surrendered to you for proper disposition.

FROM: *(Include Name, Street, City, State and ZIP Code in space provided below.)*

Signature of applicant or authorized agent
Registrant's DEA Number
Registrant's Telephone Number

NOTE: CERTIFIED MAIL (Return Receipt Requested) IS REQUIRED FOR SHIPMENTS OF DRUGS VIA U.S. POSTAL SERVICE. See instructions on reverse (page 2) of form.

	NAME OF DRUG OR PREPARATION Registrants will fill in Columns 1,2,3, and 4 ONLY.	Number of Containers	CONTENTS *(Number of grams, tablets, ounces or other units per container)*	Controlled Substance Content, *(Each Unit)*	**FOR DEA USE ONLY**		
					DISPOSITION	QUANTITY	
						GMS.	MGS.
	1	*2*	*3*	*4*	*5*	*6*	*7*
1							
2							
3							
4							
5							
6							

Figure 2–9. DEA Form 41.

A report following a multiple month study indicates that trace amounts of pharmaceuticals are present in the drinking water of 24 major U.S. metropolitan cities nationwide.[7] This problem is concerning because many pharmaceuticals maintain potency or pose toxic health threats to humans and other animals, despite water purification through rural and metropolitan treatment facilities. Although some of the contamination comes naturally through human excretion, a larger concern is the routine waste disposal of medication by consumers and pharmacies through the sewer system and landfills. In fact, pharmaceuticals are widely considered as chemical pollutants (like pesticides and industrial sewage). Drugs that affect the endocrine system (hormones), antimicrobials, and active byproducts are but a few of the pharmaceuticals found in increasing amounts in waterways and drinking water. The Environmental Protection Agency (EPA) and state health departments are expected to more rigorously enforce proper pharmaceutical disposal practices.

? Pop Quiz!

What form is required to dispose of 10 outdated morphine tubexes?

Durable and Nondurable Medical Equipment, Devices, and Supplies

Durable medical equipment, devices, and supplies are reusable products, used for the treatment of an illness or injury, that are typically ordered by a physician or other health care provider for use in a patient's place of residence. Nondurable medical equipment, devices, and supplies are manufactured for one-time use only and are disposable (Table 2-4).

Pharmacies that supply durable medical equipment, prosthetics, orthotics, and supplies can provide an important service for patients. The use of durable and nondurable medical equipment can improve a patient's quality of life. Persons with impaired mobility often use durable medical equipment. Patients who have diabetes or hypertension can self-monitor their blood glucose and blood pressure at home with medical equipment. The pharmacist can provide education for the use of medical equipment. The Centers for Medicare and Medicaid Services require that all suppliers of durable medical equipment, prosthetics, orthotics and supplies be accredited to bill Medicare Part B. As of January 1, 2010, pharmacies that supply this type of equipment must be Medicare accredited.[7] Medicare Part B covers 80% of this type of equipment and supplies. The patient must pay the 20% of the remaining cost. Persons with Medicaid can have their 20% coinsurance covered.

Many of the inventory management processes discussed in relation to pharmaceuticals also hold true for medical devices and associated supplies. One unique feature of the medical device business, however, is that some of the equipment is provided to patients on a rental or lease agreement rather than an outright purchase. In these instances, it is important that returned equipment be properly processed before being rented or leased to the next patient. Processing always includes a thorough cleaning with an approved disinfecting agent and may include sterilization of parts that come into direct contact with the patient. Between patient uses or periodically according to the manufacturer's recommendations, equipment will also undergo a biomedical review to make sure it is in proper working order, has had indicated preventive maintenance performed, and is safe for patient use. Biomedical reviews are also performed in response to reported malfunctions.

It is important to ensure that patients have the proper supplies to use with any medical equipment. Patients often need assistance in completing forms to ensure proper reimbursement related to medical devices and supplies.

It is also often necessary for a pharmacy offering medical supplies and equipment to employ staff with special training and even certifications in the fitting and use of the devices. These staff members, who may be technicians, generally assist patients in choosing the appropriate device upon a physician recommendation, help the patients ensure proper fit and match supplies to the particular device, and help educate the patients on the use of their equipment. They may also be responsible for some of the cleaning and preventive maintenance on reusable equipment.

Table 2-4. Common Durable and Nondurable Medical Equipment

Durable Medical Equipment		Nondurable Medical Equipment
Wheelchairs	Home oxygen equipment	Exam gloves
Walkers	Hospital beds	Diapers
Canes	Infusion pumps	Absorbent bed pads
Crutches	Braces	Insulin syringes and pen needles
Scooters	Blood glucose meters	Blood glucose test strips and lancets
Suction pumps	Blood pressure monitors	Dressing materials (bandages, gauze dressings, tape)
Commode and shower chairs	Nebulizers	Ostomy supplies

? Pop Quiz!

True or False? Most expired and outdated pharmaceuticals require no special disposal methods.

Suggested Reading

From *Manual for Pharmacy Technicians,* 4th ed.

Drug Distribution Processes: See Chapter 3—Ambulatory Care Pharmacy Practice; Chapter 4—Institutional Pharmacy Practice; and Chapter 5—Home Care Pharmacy Practice.

Inventory Procedures: See Chapter 19—Purchasing and Inventory Control and Chapter 2—Pharmacy Law.

Compounding and Repackaging Requirements: See Chapter 15—Nonsterile Compounding and Repackaging.

Self-Assessment Questions

1. The decision to add a drug to a hospital's formulary should always be based on which drug is cheapest to purchase.
   a. True
   b. False
2. Formulary management of inventory in hospitals and ambulatory care facilities are the same.
   a. True
   b. False
3. Which of the following is *not* a part of the normal receiving process for pharmaceuticals received from the drug wholesaler?
   a. Complete the required documentation on any investigational drugs included in the shipment.
   b. Complete the required documentation on any controlled substances included in the shipment.
   c. Verify that the box count is correct and that there are no damaged packages.
   d. Verify that all items are received and that the inventory is not expired or close to expiration.
   e. Sign and date the purchase order.
4. Provide the appropriate USP definition for each temperature.
   a. > 40° C
   b. 20° to 25° C
   c. –25° to –10° C
   d. 2° to 8° C
   e. Prevailing temperature in the work area
5. DEA form __________ must be completed upon the receipt of schedule II controlled substances.
   a. 41
   b. 227
   c. 222
   d. 106
6. Which statement is *true* regarding the placement of medications on the shelves to prevent medication errors?
   a. Generic label drugs should not be placed near the brand-name product.
   b. Look-alike drugs may be mistaken for each other and should be stored in different locations when possible.
   c. Different strengths of the same medication should never be stored next to each other because the wrong strength might be picked.
   d. The prominent placement of company logos does not contribute to medication errors and is not a factor in determining shelf placement.
   e. All of the above
7. The Pareto ABC system relies on the premise that managing 20% of your inventory will cover 80% of your costs (the 80/20 rule).
   a. True
   b. False
8. The "par-level" system of inventory management
   a. utilizes a want book to minimize ordering unnecessary pharmaceuticals
   b. uses predetermined stock minimum and maximum quantities
   c. utilizes state of the art automated perpetual inventory methods
9. Why may the FDA direct a manufacture to recall a pharmaceutical?
   a. because of contamination
   b. because of lack of potency
   c. because of lack of adherence to good manufacturing practices
   d. because of any situation that may present a significant risk to public health
   e. all of the above
10. A Class ___________ recall is the most serious of recalls; continued use of the product may result in a serious health threat or death.
    a. I
    b. II
    c. III
    d. IV
11. The IMPACT organization was formed to deal with
    a. drug recalls on a global scale
    b. pharmaceutical waste
    c. counterfeit drugs
    d. durable medical equipment

Self-Assessment Questions

12. Which of the following is *not* an example of a drug that requires special handling during receiving in the pharmacy?
    a. samples
    b. controlled substances
    c. injectables
    d. investigational drugs
    e. compounded or repackaged items
13. The DEA Form 41 is required when controlled substances are expired and need to be disposed of.
    a. True
    b. False
14. Purchasing pharmaceuticals directly from the manufacturer has more advantages to most pharmacies; as a result this is the preferred purchasing method over using a wholesaler.
    a. True
    b. False
15. Advantages of using a prime vendor contract with a wholesaler includes all of the following EXCEPT
    a. more timely ordering and delivery
    b. fewer inventory carrying costs
    c. the pharmacy needs a large storage capacity
    d. less documentation
    e. supports the "just-in-time" philosophy
16. The intent of the RDDS is to insure
    a. the specific drugs identified as high risk are safely procured, prescribed, dispensed, and administered
    b. chemotherapy drugs are safely procured, prescribed, dispensed, and administered
    c. chemotherapy drugs are safely wasted and disposed of
17. RDDS drugs can cause serious adverse health reactions such as
    a. ototoxicity
    b. blood disorders and birth defects
    c. nausea and vomiting
    d. hepatoxicity
18. In most cases RDDS requires documentation of
    1.
    2.
    3.
    4.
    5.
    6.
19. Reusable medical devices must be
    a. cleaned between patient uses
    b. checked between uses to ensure that they are functioning properly
    c. maintained with all manufacturer-recommended preventive maintenance
    d. tested for proper function in response to any report of malfunction
    e. all of the above
20. _________ is disposable.
    a. Durable medical equipment
    b. Nondurable medical equipment

Self-Assessment Answers

1. b
2. b
3. a
4. excessive heat; controlled room temperature; freezer; refrigerated; room temperature
5. b
6. b
7. a
8. b
9. e
10. a
11. c
12. c
13. a
14. b
15. c
16. a
17. a
18. 1. Registration of prescribing physician, 2. Dispensing pharmacy, 3. Patient name and other demographic information, 4. Patient agreement for liability purposes, 5. Specific indication for medication, 6. Dose and quantity dispensed
19. e
20. b

Chapter 3

Administration and Management of Pharmacy Practice

Learning Outcomes

After completing this chapter, the technician should be able to:

- Define the benefits of joint commission accreditation and certification.
- Give examples of policies and procedures relating to the practice of pharmacy.
- Differentiate between quality control and continuous quality improvement mechanisms.
- List the elements required by federal law to be on a prescription label.
- List exemptions to the Poison Prevention Packaging Act.
- Discuss special handling requirements for controlled substances.
- Discuss the regulatory authority of state boards of pharmacy.
- Discuss the elements of effective communication utilized in pharmacy practice including oral, written, and electronic means of communication.
- State the intent of the Omnibus Budget Reconciliation Act of 1990 (OBRA 90) and describe the requirements it mandates.
- State the intent of the Health Insurance Portability and Accountability Act of 1996 (HIPAA) and describe the requirements it mandates.
- Discuss pharmacy record-keeping requirements.
- Discuss the rules and regulations governing billing and reimbursement procedures.
- Describe the correct procedures for cleaning and maintaining equipment used in compounding.

This chapter applies to Section III of the PTCB exam, Participating in the Administration and Management of Pharmacy Practice.

Pharmacy Operations

Pharmacy technicians play an integral role in the daily operation of pharmacy services in both community and hospital practice settings. They must know the regulations for regulatory agencies, standards utilized for scheduled drugs, and the rules and regulations that govern billing and reimbursement. This chapter will serve to familiarize you with many of the normal operation procedures for pharmacy practice.

Preparing for Accrediting and Regulatory Agency Visits

Regulatory and accrediting agencies make site visits to inspect and verify that their published standards of care are being met. They meet with health care providers to determine how patients are being cared for in the institution. As part of this site visit, the evaluation team may review documented guidelines and policy and procedure manuals. The preparation for the site visits is frequently a multidisciplinary effort in which technicians often participate as a key member on the health care team.

One of the most recognized accrediting agencies for hospitals is The Joint Commission (TJC; formerly known as the Joint Commission on the Accreditation of Healthcare Organizations, or JCAHO). The Joint Commission is an independent, not-for-profit organization that accredits and certifies more than 15,000 health care organizations and programs in the United States. It publishes guides and checklists on how to prepare for on-site inspections. Pharmacy technicians need to be familiar with and trained on these published requirements and standards.

The benefits of Joint Commission accreditation and certification include:

- strengthening community confidence in the quality and safety of care, treatment, and services
- providing a competitive edge in the marketplace
- improving risk management and risk reduction
- providing education on good practices to improve business operations
- providing professional advice and counsel, enhancing staff education
- enhancing staff recruitment and development
- recognition by select insurers and other third parties
- fulfillment of regulatory requirements in select states

Policies and Procedures

Policies and procedures (P&P) are documents that provide guidance about expectations of the behavior of employees of the hospital, business, or pharmacy department. General P&P cover areas such as hiring requirements and employee benefits. Pharmacy P&P cover issues concerning the delivery of efficient, quality drug therapy, including the following:

- correct aseptic (sterile) technique when compounding intravenous (IV) admixtures
- good compounding practices
- repackaging processes
- monitoring patients for drug allergies
- proper handling of cancer chemotherapeutic agents
- distribution and control of all drugs used in the organization
- procedures for ensuring that patients receive the correct drugs
- use of investigational (experimental) drugs
- management of toxic or dangerous drugs
- provision of pharmacy services in the event of a disaster
- identification of medications brought into the organization by patients
- management of drug expenditures and the pharmacy budget
- staffing levels
- identification of prescription forgeries and theft prevention strategies
- billing procedures and maintenance of customer accounts
- inventory control and maintenance procedures
- management of medical equipment

Many accrediting organizations, such as the Joint Commission (TJC; formerly known as the Joint Commission on the Accreditation of Healthcare Organizations, or JCAHO), and professional organizations, such as the American Society of Health-System Pharmacists (ASHP), require that pharmacy departments develop and maintain P&P manuals. Pharmacy department P&P are developed by the director of pharmacy or the pharmacist-in-charge or owner in a retail establishment (or by corporate headquarters for a chain store). These documents are generally revised and updated annually and are compiled in a readily available manual or kept available online for easy access by all employees.

Quality Assurance Mechanisms

Quality control and continuous quality improvement (CQI) programs are also required by many of the accrediting agencies, such as the JTC and the Centers for Medicare and Medicaid Services (CMS; formerly the Health Care Financing Administration, or HCFA). Quality improvement is good practice, even if it is not required by regulatory oversight. The following are just a few examples of quality control and quality improvement activities:

- completing refrigerator temperature logs
- documenting inspections of nursing units and other medication stock areas
- decreasing legibility errors by working with local physicians to provide electronic prescription transmission
- improving medication turnaround time in the hospital by automating dispensing
- decreasing wrong-drug/wrong-patient errors through the use of bar code identification systems
- updating patient files at each prescription encounter to ensure that patient information is correct

Quality can be ensured through the use of quality control and through continuous quality improvement methods.

Quality Control

Quality control is a set of procedures followed during the manufacturing of a product or provision of a service to ensure that the end product or service meets or exceeds specified standards. Checks and balances usually occur at critical points in the process. The start of any quality control program requires complete written procedures and training for all staff members involved in that procedure. Although quality control identifies and prevents errors or defects, it does not always identify or correct the underlying cause.

Quality Improvement

Quality improvement (QI) is a scientific and systematic process involving monitoring, evaluating, and identifying problems and developing and measuring the impact of the improvement strategies. It requires that decisions be based on facts (data).There are numerous QI models used today, including Six Sigma, Zero Defects, Total Quality Management (TQM), and Continuous Quality Improvement (CQI).[16] There are also many tools used to identify problems, collect data, and analyze data. An example of a tool involving statistics is a run chart, which tracks patterns and trends over a period of time.

Technicians play key roles in many of the performance-improvement activities such as participating on performance improvement teams to collect and analyze data. Technicians may also assist in database management for quality improvement services such as adverse drug reaction reports, medication error reports, and medication use evaluations.

Medication safety is an emphasis in all areas of pharmacy; it is at the heart of all processes involving and applying performance improvement.

? Pop Quiz!

What is one of the most recognized accreditation agencies?

Compliance with Federal and State Law

Although states have the primary authority to regulate pharmacy practice, pharmacy is also subject to a number of federal laws. Examples of federal laws include:

- Food, Drug, and Cosmetic Act (FDCA)
- The Controlled Substances Act
- The Omnibus Budget Reconciliation Act of 1990

Prescription Label Requirements

The FDCA requires that all retail prescription labels have the following information:

- name and address of pharmacy
- prescription number
- date of prescription filling or refilling
- name of prescriber
- name of patient
- directions for use
- cautionary statement (as indicated on the prescription)

Medication orders in long-term care facilities and hospitals are different from retail prescriptions; therefore, the labels do not require the same information. Labels on medicines in long-term care facilities or hospitals may not include quantity dispensed, cautionary statements, original filling date, prescriber's name, or even the name and address of the pharmacy. Most states have rules for what must appear on prescription or medication order labels. Therefore, the technician should review the state's rules regarding labeling.

Prescription Refill Requirements

A prescription can usually be refilled as many times as the prescriber indicates on the prescription, within a time period determined by the state. This time period is usually 1 year from the date the prescription was written. If the number of refills does not appear on the prescription, it is assumed that refills are not authorized.

Patients who do not have refills on a prescription may request that the pharmacist ask the prescriber to authorize refills. An emergency supply of medication, usually not more than a 72-hour supply, may be dispensed to a patient if the pharmacist is unable to obtain refill authorization and determines that the patient may suffer harm if a lapse in therapy occurs.

Poison Prevention Packaging Act

The Poison Prevention Packaging Act was enacted to reduce the number of poisonings in children from drugs and chemicals. The law requires that all prescriptions and most over-the-counter drugs be dispensed in containers with child-resistant closures, unless the drug or container falls under one of the many exceptions. These child-resistant prescription containers cannot be reused for refills. This law usually applies to retail settings. It does not apply to the dispensing of prescriptions to inpatients in long-term care facilities or hospitals, but it does apply to prescriptions dispensed to those patients upon discharge. Therefore, when filling a prescription for a patient who is being discharged from the institution to return home, the drug must be dispensed in a container with a child-resistant closure.

Some drugs, such as nitroglycerin, oral contraceptives, and other drugs packaged for patient use by the manufacturer (such as prepackaged methylprednisolone) do not require the child-resistant container. The list, with exceptions, of drugs that require safety closures is available from the U.S. Consumer Product Safety Commission's Web site, http://www.cpsc.gov/CPSCPUB/PUBS/384.pdf.

Because many patients do not have children at home or may have a disease that impairs their ability to open child-resistant containers, the patient, caregiver, or physician may request that the prescription be dispensed in a non-child-resistant container. Federal law does not require a written request to have the prescription dispensed in a non-child-resistant container. However, physicians who make this request must do so on a patient-by-patient basis and not in the form of a blanket request for all or a group of patients.

? Pop Quiz!

Give two examples of medications that are exempt from the Poison Prevention Packaging Act.

Prescription Drug Information for Patients

Pharmacists provide patients with different types of written information for their prescription drugs. Patients are provided with printed information about their **dispensed medication** called *consumer medication information* or *CMI.* In addition, the FDA requires pharmacists to provide patients with *patient package insert ("PPI")* with the dispensing of certain prescription drugs such as estrogens and oral contraceptives.

Controlled Substance Regulations

The Federal Controlled Substance Act was enacted to protect the public by controlling the flow of dangerous drugs into the community. The United States Department of Justice Drug Enforcement Agency (DEA) takes responsibility for vigilance over the distribution of these drugs in research, institutions, and the community. This agency plays an important role in creating the rules that govern the practice of pharmacy.

Drugs that are watched by the DEA are called *controlled substances.* Controlled substances are divided into five categories, or schedules. Schedule I drugs are substances with a high abuse potential and no legitimate medical purpose. Schedule II drugs are those with high abuse potential and a recognized medical purpose. Schedules III, IV, and V drugs have legitimate medical purpose but less abuse potential. For all practical purposes, Schedules III, IV, and V drugs are treated the same from a regulatory perspective.

To order a prescription for a controlled substance, the prescriber must be registered with the Department of Justice and be issued a DEA registration number. Similarly, to dispense a controlled substance, a pharmacy must have a DEA registration number.

Schedules of Controlled Substances

Schedule II

Some examples of single-entity Schedule II narcotics include morphine, codeine, hydrocodone, and opium. Other Schedule II narcotic substances and their common name-brand products include hydromorphone (Dilaudid®), methadone (Dolophine®), meperidine (Demerol®), oxycodone (Percodan®), and fentanyl (Sublimaze®). Some examples of Schedule II stimulants include amphetamine (Dexedrine®, Adderall®), methamphetamine (Desoxyn®), and methylphenidate (Ritalin®). Other Schedule II substances include cocaine, amobarbital, glutethimide, pentobarbital, and secobarbital.

Schedule III

Some examples of Schedule III narcotics include products containing less than 15 milligrams of hydrocodone per dosage unit (Vicodin®, Lorcet®, Tussionex®) and products containing not more than 90 milligrams of codeine per dosage unit (codeine with acetaminophen, aspirin, or ibuprofen). Other Schedule III substances include anabolic steroids, benzphetamine (Didrex®), phendimetrazine, and any compound, mixture, preparation, or suppository dosage form containing amobarbital, secobarbital, pentobarbital, dronabinol (Marinol®), or ketamine.

Schedule IV

The substances in this schedule have an abuse potential less than those in Schedule III and more than those in Schedule V. Some examples of Schedule IV narcotics include propoxyphene (Darvon®), butorphanol (Stadol®), and pentazocine (Talwin-NX®). The following benzodiazepine substances are also found in Schedule IV: alprazolam (Xanax®), clonazepam (Klonopin®), clorazepate (Tranxene®), diazepam (Valium®), flurazepam (Dalmane®), halazepam (Paxipam®), lorazepam (Ativan®), midazolam (Versed®), oxazepam (Serax®), prazepam (Centrax®), temazepam (Restoril®), triazolam (Halcion®), and quazepam (Doral®). Other Schedule IV substances include barbital, phenobarbital, chloral hydrate, ethchlorvynol (Placidyl®), chlordiazepoxide (Librium®), ethinamate, meprobamate, paraldehyde, methohexital, phentermine, diethylpropion, pemoline (Cylert®), mazindol (Sanorex®), and sibutramine (Meridia®).

Schedule V

The substances in this schedule have an abuse potential less than those in Schedule IV and consist primarily of preparations containing limited quantities of certain narcotic and stimulant drugs, generally for antitussive, antidiarrheal, or analgesic purposes. Some examples are cough preparations containing not more than 200 milligrams of codeine per 100 milliliters or per 100 grams (Robitussin AC®, Phenergan with Codeine®) and buprenorphine (Buprenex®).

List I Chemicals

In addition to Schedules I through V controlled substances, the DEA monitors List I and List II chemicals. These are chemicals that can be used in the synthesis of other chemicals that are controlled substances. The pharmacy must account for List I and List II chemicals. Pseudoephedrine is a common List I chemical. The use of these chemicals in compounding may have to be reported to the DEA, depending on a state's rules.

States also will place certain drugs into a schedule. Occasionally, a conflict arises when a state and the federal government do not agree on which schedule a drug should be. If such a conflict arises, the stricter scheduling will apply.

State Boards of Pharmacy

State pharmacy laws establish the legal requirements, restrictions, and prohibitions for the practice of pharmacy. State laws are enacted by state legislatures through the legislative process. If the state and federal laws or regulations differ, both laws and regulations must be followed, including the more stringent requirement whether state or federal.

Pharmacy technician requirements vary from state to state; however, an important and universal distinction for pharmacy technicians to understand is that they work under the supervision and direction of the pharmacist and may only perform the tasks that are permitted under State Law. State pharmacy laws do not permit pharmacy technicians to perform pharmacy tasks and responsibilities that are limited to pharmacists and require the professional judgment, education, and training of a pharmacist.

State boards of pharmacy are responsible for regulating the practice of pharmacy, including pharmacies, pharmacists, pharmacy interns, and pharmacy technicians. The state boards of pharmacy have regulatory authority over a number of areas, such as:

- licensing pharmacies and pharmacists
- registering or licensing pharmacy technicians
- inspecting pharmacies
- issuing rules and regulations
- investigating complaints, and disciplinary actions against pharmacies, pharmacists, and pharmacy technicians for violations of pharmacy laws and regulations

State boards of pharmacy have also enacted regulations pertaining to patient counseling by pharmacists. Information on the various state boards of pharmacy is available through the National Association of Boards of Pharmacy (NABP) Web site at www.nabp.net.

? Pop Quiz!

Codeine is an example of what kind of controlled substance?

Counseling Requirements

The Omnibus Reconciliation Act of 1990 (OBRA 90) required states that receive federal funding to create programs to improve the quality of pharmaceutical care and save money by educating patients on the proper use of drugs. The program required pharmacists to obtain certain information from the patient, including personal identifying information, disease state, medication allergies, and other information that would be important for determining proper drug therapy. This federal program targeted only Medicaid and Medicare patients, but most states expanded it to include all patients.

Although most states require the pharmacist to provide the counseling, the pharmacy technician's role in this program is important in obtaining information from the patient. The pharmacy technician should ask patients if they desire counseling for all prescription products in addition to any OTC products the patient is purchasing.

OBRA 90 further mandated that pharmacists provide counseling for individuals or their caregivers. The pharmacist or a designee must extend an offer for medication counseling to the patient. The offer may be written or oral. The pharmacist must always perform the actual counseling session. The patient may decline counseling, and if so, this should be documented.

OBRA 90 and most state counseling regulations require that the following eight areas be covered in patient counseling:

- the name and description of the medication
- the route of administration, dosage, and dosage form
- special directions and precautions for preparation, administration, and use by the patient
- common severe side effects, adverse effects, interactions, and therapeutic contraindications
- techniques for self-monitoring therapy
- proper storage
- prescription refill information
- action to be taken in the case of a missed dose

Record-Keeping Requirements

The FDCA describes the records that pharmacists are required to keep. One of the main reasons pharmacists are required to record the receipt, disposition, and accountability of drugs is to ensure that the pharmacy can contact patients who received a drug that has been recalled.

Purchase invoices are records of drug receipt, prescriptions are records of drug disposition, and inventories provide a record of drugs in stock. Some type of written document should evidence any sales, disposals, returns, destruction, or theft of drugs. Rules vary as to the length of time records must be kept, but in general, it should not be less than 5 years. Some states may require longer storage of certain records.

The Health Insurance Portability and Accountability Act of 1996 (HIPAA)

The Health Insurance Portability and Accountability Act of 1996 (HIPAA) has strengthened patient privacy rights. Although this was not the only purpose of the law, the pharmacy's role in maintaining confidentiality has also increased. Patient records must be guarded from disclosure to unauthorized individuals and companies. Pharmacy employees are prohibited from discussing a patient's medical history except for purposes relevant to the patient's care. All written information concerning a patient should be discarded in such a manner as to protect the patient's identity. Utilizing shredders or professional document disposal services is now common pharmacy practice. Pharmacy technicians should only discuss information regarding the patient's therapy so that unauthorized persons will not overhear such discussions. Technicians should also be aware that using overhead paging systems to announce a patient's name could undermine a patient's privacy. Most pharmacies will have policies and procedures in place to address the requirements of HIPAA.

Communication and Teamwork

It is important for pharmacy technicians to develop effective communication skills to help strengthen professional relationships and ensure an appropriate information exchange. These skills will enable the pharmacy technician to better assist the pharmacist in providing patient-centered care and manage pharmacy operations.

Pharmacists are involved in patient-centered communication, the responsible provision of drug therapy for the purpose of achieving definite outcomes that improve a patient's quality of life.

Pharmacy technicians play an important role in the patient's safe use of medication. Often the pharmacy technician is the first person that the patient encounters. Appropriate appearance, behavior, professionalism, knowledge, and communication skills of the technician cannot be overemphasized.

Verbal communication is the most common form of interpersonal communication. It involves a spoken message delivered from a sender to a recipient. Nonverbal communication is the exchange of messages by means other than speaking. This may include, but is not limited to, appearance and behavior, body language, physical distance, and physical contact.

Body language can be interpreted as unconsciously conveying one's feelings or psychological state of mind and can have a profound impact on how the message is received by the recipient. Inappropriate expressions such as lack of eye contact or rolling of the eyes should be avoided. Body postures that convey attention and interest should be used rather than the using of a closed posture showing a lack of interest.

Telephone encounters are a high percentage of the communication contacts made by a pharmacy technician on a daily basis. Nonverbal skills are not as significant but still play a role. Clearly, how the message is spoken impacts how the message is perceived by the recipient. At the beginning of the telephone conversation the pharmacy technician should identify themselves by name and title as well as the name of the pharmacy or department.

Internet and Electronic Communication

The use of the Internet and facsimile (fax) for communications has greatly expanded in pharmacy practice settings. The principles of effective written communication should be followed.

Never ask patients to provide information over the Internet that could lead to "identity theft" unless it is transmitted through the use of a security-encrypted Web site. When faxing documents, be sure to include a cover sheet to ensure the complete information reaches the appropriate person and follow the Health Insurance Portability and Accountability Act (HIPAA) requirements to maintain the privacy of patient protected health information (PHI). For important documents, use a method of verification of information receipt.

Teamwork

Pharmacy technicians are members of the healthcare team. They have a responsibility to promote the principles of the team. This can be done by the following behaviors:

- cultivating trust and confidence among team members
- recognizing the contributions of all team members
- working with other team members to solve problems and develop ideas
- minimizing politics by respecting professional boundaries
- helping to align the team around the common objectives and priorities
- establishing respect and appreciation among team members
- holding oneself and other team members to the same high standards
- putting the team's goals ahead of personal interests and goals

It is also the responsibility of team members to identify and disclose unprofessional behaviors among team members, which could jeopardize the team and the services provided. In pharmacy settings, these situations (eg, medication errors, drug diversion, substance abuse impairment, patient discrimination or harassment, theft, etc.) could result in negative effects on services, operations, and patient health. The pharmacy technician should play an active role in the detection and prevention of these issues by bringing irregularities to the attention of the pharmacist or appropriate supervisory personnel.

Billing and Reimbursement

Pharmacy Reimbursement Basics

One of the most time-consuming activities in the ambulatory care pharmacy setting is dealing with third party payment programs. Reimbursement for pharmaceuticals is complex and widely variable. Most prescription plans allow for "on-line adjudication" of prescriptions. This process verifies the patient's eligibility, identifies the reimbursement type, and identifies any fee due from the patient at the time of purchase. The exact methodology that is used to bill and reimburse for drugs will vary based upon several factors, including:

- the practice setting in which the drug is dispensed
- the type of drug that is being dispensed
- who is paying for the drug

In community pharmacy practice, the most common type of payment method is retrospective or **fee for service**. In the **retrospective payment** model, drugs are dispensed and later reimbursed according to a predetermined formula that is specified in a contract between the pharmacy and the **third party payer,** such as the insurance company or pharmacy benefit manager. The reimbursement rate for third party prescriptions is based on a formula consisting of various parts: ingredient cost, dispensing fee, and patient copayments. The ingredient cost is the amount paid to the pharmacy for the cost of the drug product, the **dispensing fee** is an amount paid for dispensing the prescription, and the **copayment** (also known as "copay") is the cost-sharing amount paid by the patient or customer.

- Third party reimbursement = (ingredient cost + dispensing fee) – copayment

Historically, the average wholesale price (AWP) has been the most commonly used benchmark used for billing drugs that are reimbursed in the community pharmacy setting. AWP is usually set at 20–25% above the wholesale acquisition cost (WAC). Wholesale acquisition cost (WAC) is set by each manufacturer. It represents the "list price" at which the manufacturer sells the drug to the wholesaler. There is growing recognition that neither AWP nor WAC represents what is actually paid for drugs.

New benchmarks that are used for drug pricing within the past decade include average sales price (ASP) and average manufacturer price (AMP). ASP is based on manufacturer reported selling price data and includes volume discounts and price concessions that are offered to all classes of trade. AMP is the average price paid to manufacturers by wholesalers for drugs distributed through retail pharmacies. AMP includes discounts and other price concessions that are provided by manufacturers. AMP was created by Congress in 1990 to facilitate calculating Medicaid rebates. The Budget Deficit Reduction Act of 2005 (DRA) requires that AMP be used to calculate the **federal upper limit (FUL)** for drugs that are paid through Medicaid. The FUL represents the maximum of federal matching funds the federal government will pay to state Medicaid programs for eligible generic and multi-source drugs. With the enactment of the Patient Protection and Affordable Care Act of 2010 (health care reform) on March 23, 2010, the AMP was established as 175% of the ASP.

Typically, the reimbursement formula for a generic product is different than for a brand product. Sole source or brand-name drugs are usually reimbursed based upon AWP or WAC, whereas generic or multi-source drugs are reimbursed based upon a **maximum allowable cost (MAC)** schedule, which is usually based upon the cost of the lowest available generic equivalent.

Sample formulas:

- sole source drug reimbursement = AWP – 15% + $3.50 dispensing fee
- multi-source drug reimbursement = MAC + $3.50 dispensing fee

Payment for Drugs and Pharmacy Services

Self-Pay

Although many patients have some form of prescription drug coverage, a significant number are still uninsured or underinsured. The amount that is paid by a cash-paying customer is often referred to as the "usual and customary price" or the "cash price." Many third party contracts will indicate that the amount to be paid for a prescription is based upon a reimbursement formula (as explained above) or the usual and customary price. The lower of the two prices is the amount usually paid.

Many drug companies offer certain free drugs through **patient assistance programs (PAPs)** to low-income patients who lack prescription drug coverage and meet certain criteria. Some companies also offer bulk replacement or **institutional patient assistance programs (IPAP)**. In the IPAP model, medications are provided to an institution (eg, pharmacy or clinic) rather than to the individual patient. The 340B drug-pricing program is another option that can be utilized to assist patients who lack adequate prescription drug coverage. There are several types of facilities that qualify as "covered entities" for 340B pricing, including federal qualified health centers (FQHC), disproportionate share hospitals (DSH) and state-owned AIDS drug assistance programs. The Office of Pharmacy Affairs, which is located within Health Resources and Services Administration, administers the 340B drug discount program.

Private Insurance

Private insurance can be either managed care (based on a network of providers) or indemnity (non-network based coverage). Managed care is a type of private health insurance or health care organization that is based on networks of providers, such as pharmacies, doctors, and hospitals. **Indemnity** insurance offers more choices of physicians and hospitals, but the employee's out-of-pocket costs are higher than with managed care.

Pharmacy Benefit Managers

Pharmacy benefit managers (PBM) are organizations that administer pharmacy benefits for private or public third party payers, also known as plan sponsors. These organizations may include managed care organizations, self-insured employers, insurance companies, labor unions, Medicaid and Medicare prescription drug plans, the Federal Employees Health Benefits Program, and other federal, state, and local government entities. A plan sponsor chooses a PBM to manage the pharmacy benefit; the sponsor pays the PBM a fee that is usually based on the number of beneficiaries (plan members and dependents) who are covered by the pharmacy benefit. The fee should cover the total cost of the pharmacy benefit (including all prescriptions) for the covered beneficiaries. The PBM designs and manages the pharmacy benefit so that the cost of prescriptions dispensed does not exceed the amount of money paid to the PBM by the sponsor.

The **formulary** is the cornerstone of any PBM's activities. It is a specific list of drugs that is included with a given pharmacy benefit. The formulary usually includes both brand and generic drugs in most therapeutic categories. Brand name drugs can be either preferred (designated by the PBM as the first-choice drugs) or non-preferred. The PBM may charge different copays for different types of formulary drugs.

The PBM can utilize administrative tools within the context of the formulary in order to optimize the clinical and economic performance of the pharmacy benefit. Some of the more common administrative tools are prior authorization, step therapy, and quantity limits.

- **Prior authorization** requires the prescriber to receive preapproval from the PBM in order for the drug to be covered by the benefit.
- **Step therapy** requires use of a recognized first-line drug before a more complex or expensive second-line drug is used.
- **Quantity limits** set upper limits of the amount of a drug that will be covered by the benefit, or the total days of therapy.

Processing Private Third Party Prescriptions

Patients with a prescription drug benefit should have a prescription identification (ID) card. The information on the prescription ID card is necessary in order to submit a claim to the PBM.

The card will identify the PBM (any PBM) or drug benefit provider. It will show a telephone number for the PBM's customer service department. The employer may be identified (Your Company, Inc.), followed by the member name (Jane Doe) and member ID number (12345678). If the beneficiary is different from the plan member, such as a dependent child, the participant's name may be listed. Finally, the BIN # (000012) is the bank identification number, which is also needed to submit the claim. It references the claims processor or PBM.

Once the technician enters information in the pharmacy computer from the prescription ID card and the prescription, the PBM will either accept or reject the claim. If the claim is rejected, the PBM will respond with a message, commonly known as a rejection code. The technician must assess the meaning of the rejection code and respond accordingly. If the issue cannot be resolved, the technician may need to place a call to the PBM to resolve the issue.

Public Payers

Medicare

Medicare is the federal health program for the elderly, disabled, and people with end-stage renal disease or amyotrophic lateral sclerosis (ALS). Most people automatically qualify for Medicare once they turn 65 and are eligible for Social Security payments, and if they or their spouse have made payroll tax contributions to Medicare for a total of 10 years or 40 quarters. There are four parts to Medicare:

- Part A (hospital insurance)
- Part B (medical insurance)
- Part C (Medicare Advantage plans)
- Part D (prescription drug coverage)

Medicare Part A

Medicare Part A helps cover inpatient care (hospitals, skilled nursing facilities, hospice care, and some home health care). For most people, Part A coverage is prepaid through payroll taxes. Medicare Part A coverage involves a **deductible** and a benefit period of 60 days. A deductible is an out-of-pocket amount that must be paid before insurance coverage begins. Full Medicare coverage applies for the first 60 days; thereafter, the beneficiary is responsible for **coinsurance**, which is a fixed percentage charge for a service. Part A claims are processed by a fiscal intermediary, and the **diagnosis-related group (DRG)** is the basis for reimbursement.

Medicare Part B

Medicare Part B is optional medical insurance for outpatient physician and hospital services, clinical laboratory services, and durable medical equipment, prosthetics, orthotics, and supplies (DMEPOS). Part B coverage involves paying a monthly premium, an annual deductible, and coinsurance.

Medicare Part C

Medicare Part C is the Medicare Advantage Plan, which combines Part A and B coverage. Under this plan, benefits are provided by Medicare-approved private insurance companies. These private fee-for-service and managed care plans often include prescription drug benefits, called Medicare Advantage Prescription Drug plans or MAPDs; as such, Part C beneficiaries should not enroll in a Part D prescription drug plan. There are five types of Part C plans:

- health maintenance organizations (HMO)
- preferred provider organizations (PPO)
- medical savings account plans

- private fee-for-service plans
- Medicare special needs plans

Medicare Advantage Plans charge one combined premium for Part A and B benefits and prescription drug coverage (if included in the plan).

Medicare Part D

Medicare Part D is a federal prescription drug program that is paid for by the Centers for Medicare and Medicaid Services (CMS) and by individual premiums. It was enacted as part of the Medicare Prescription Drug, Improvement, and Modernization Act of 2003. Medicare Part D offers a voluntary insurance benefit for outpatient prescription drugs. Medicare prescription drug plans are administered by private PBMs or other companies approved by Medicare. Each plan varies in terms of cost and drugs covered. Drug formularies for Medicare Part D vary from plan to plan. CMS requires that all Medicare prescription drug plans cover at least two drugs in each therapeutic category. There are six categories of drugs that must include almost all drugs in the category due to the importance of the therapeutic class and the need for beneficiaries to have access to all drugs in the class. The six protected drug categories are:

- antipsychotics
- antidepressants
- antiepileptics
- immunosuppressants
- cancer
- HIV/AIDS drugs

There are some classes of drugs that are not covered at all by Medicare Part D. These are:

- over-the-counter drugs
- benzodiazepines
- barbiturates
- drugs for weight loss or weight gain
- drugs for erectile dysfunction.

Processing Medicare Part D prescriptions is similar to processing prescriptions from any other private insurance company or PBM. All Part D claims must contain a National Provider Identifier (NPI). If the prescriber does not have an NPI, or if the pharmacy cannot locate the prescriber's NPI, a non-NPI prescriber ID can be submitted on the claim if allowed by the payer.

Medicaid

Medicaid is a medical and long-term care program that is jointly funded by the federal and state governments. Participation in Medicaid is optional for states; however, since 1982, all states participate in the Medicaid program. Medicaid covers three main groups of low-income Americans: parents and children, the elderly, and the disabled. Patients whose incomes exceed the established guidelines for eligibility may qualify for Medicaid if they have medical expenses that exceed a certain threshold. This type of coverage is commonly known as "spend down." As explained above, the Medicare Prescription Drug benefit, which provides prescription drug coverage for qualified senior citizens, was implemented in January 2006. Medicaid recipients who also qualify for Medicare are known as "dual eligible." Medicare is usually considered the primary payer for medical benefits for dual eligible patients; however, Medicaid can supplement Medicare benefits by providing coverage for benefits that may not be covered by Medicare and/or providing assistance with copayments for prescription medications. Medicaid functions as the "safety net" or payer of last resort.

In addition to Medicare and Medicaid, the government pays for health benefit programs for the Department of Veterans Affairs, Department of Defense, and the Indian Health Service. All veterans of active military service (Army, Navy, Air Force, Marines, and Coast Guard) are potentially eligible for health benefits from the Department of Veterans Affairs.

Claims Processing

Billing Methods in Institutional Pharmacy

Most billing in institutional settings is imbedded within the patient's overall bill for the stay. Separate payments are not made for drugs; the drug costs are included in the diagnosis-related groups (DRG), which are used to determine the payments made to the hospital by insurers. DRG were introduced in the early 1980s as part of a prospective payment system (PPS) to classify hospital cases based primarily on type of patient, diagnoses, procedures, complications, comorbidities, and resources used. Patients admitted for a hospital stay are assigned a DRG. Payment or reimbursement for inpatient services are often predetermined and are based on this DRG-based prospective payment system. There are three basic systems: billing at the time of order entry, billing at the time of dispensing, and billing at the time of administration.

Billing at the time of order entry charges the dispensed quantity of medication to the patient as soon as the order is entered by the pharmacy. Subsequent charges are transmitted every time the order is refilled for the patient. Some order entry charges assume a "flat rate charge" for the use or availability of the medication. A flat rate might occur, for example, on an order for a sliding scale insulin, rather than a charge for each administration. The flat rate is generally based on average usage for the order type.

Billing at the time of dispensing is a common method in many institutions that use point-of-care dispensing technology, such as Omnicell® or Pyxis®. The medication, rather than being charged at the time of order entry, is charged when withdrawn from the machine. This system may make billing more accurate by eliminating charges for lost medications. It also eliminates a lot of the crediting activity created when medications are returned to the pharmacy unused after being billed at the time of order entry.

Billing at the time of administration is the most accurate and efficient of the three. This system can be used when bedside bar code recognition of the patient and the medication allows for billing to be transmitted by the bar code reader.

Billing Methods in Outpatient and Clinic Settings

In an outpatient hospital, clinic, or physician office setting, physician-administered drugs may either be included as part of the procedure or paid separately. Most drugs given in this setting are considered fee-for-service or separately billable (if the drug exceeds the Medicare packaging threshold). Typically, the fee-for-service formula is based on AWP. Some drugs are bundled into the ambulatory payment classification (APC). APCs are pre-determined outpatient payment categories, similar to inpatient DRGs.

Each drug charge requires the appropriate **Healthcare Common Procedure Coding System (HCPCS)** code, and the quantity should be billed in service unit increments. Service units are pre-determined billing increments that may be unrelated to the package size.

Key data elements necessary for claim submission include:

- beneficiary name and Health Insurance Claim Number (HICN)
- date of service
- Healthcare Common Procedure Code System (HCPCS) codes
- Common Procedural Terminology (CPT) codes
- International Classification of Diseases, 9th Revision (ICD-9) codes (also known as Diagnosis codes)
- clinical modifiers
- National Drug Code (NDC)
- units of service (quantity expressed in service units or billing increments)
- place of service

Community Pharmacy

The majority of pharmacy claims are submitted by community pharmacies and reimbursed by a third party payer. When working in the outpatient care setting, it is essential to understand how drugs are billed and paid. The prescription drug claims **adjudication** process involves the following steps:

- submitting appropriate information
- determining eligibility, coverage, and payment
- communicating reimbursement
- settling the claim

Today, the pharmacy industry uses the NCPDP Telecommunications Standard Format Version 5.1 to adjudicate prescription drug claims through the electronic, online, real-time system. The system was created to standardize the exchange of data for claims submission and adjudication. This format allows communication of claims between pharmacy providers, pharmacy benefit managers, third party payers, and insurance carriers at the point of service. Pharmacy technicians can verify eligibility, determine formulary coverage status, confirm quantity limits and copay amounts, submit claims, and receive payment information.

Prescription Processing

In order to submit an electronic on-line claim, key billing elements include:

- prescription processor (insurance company or contracted PBM information on the ID card)
- BIN (bank identification number)
    - PCN (processor control number)

- pharmacy provider information (specific to each pharmacy)
  - NPI (National Provider Identification) – effective May 23, 2008
  - NCPDP or NABP (formerly NPIC = National Pharmacy Identification Code)
- eligibility (specific to each patient)
  - member name and identification number (unique identifier)
  - group number (insurers have several groups or plans)
  - relationship (plan member, spouse, dependent)
- prescription information
  - date of prescription (date when prescription was written and each fill)
  - NDC = National Drug Code (which identifies the manufacturer, drug, strength, dosage form, and package size)
  - directions for use
  - quantity dispensed
  - days supply
  - refills (number of refills authorized)
  - Dispense as Written (DAW) or product substitution
  - physician signature (electronic signature, if permitted), NPI number, and DEA number, when required

In a community pharmacy setting, prescription claims are submitted online and adjudicated in real time. Although the computer software offers guidance for correct billing practices, it cannot prevent all errors. Outlined below are basic elements and pharmacy procedures used to enter prescription-billing information.

Information necessary to file a claim is available on the prescription drug ID card and includes the following:

- cardholder ID
- group number
- dependent coverage (relationship codes)
  - 1 = cardholder or eligible primary person or subscriber
  - 2 = spouse of cardholder
  - 3 = dependent child
  - 4 = other (eg, disabled dependent, dependent adult, dependent parent, domestic partner)
- BIN and PCN numbers

Audits

Pharmacies are often subject to audits by third party payers, which can result in situations in which pharmacies are required to pay back third party payers.

? Pop Quiz!

A prescription says one tablet q 12 h. How many must be dispensed for a 10-day course of therapy?

Maintenance of Pharmacy Equipment

Cross-contamination resulting from microbes or drug product residue on equipment and work surfaces will not occur if written policies regarding cleaning and maintenance are followed and documented. Most automatic, mechanical, electronic, or other types of equipment have written programs for maintenance and cleaning to ensure proper performance. Technicians should familiarize themselves with these programs and document that these procedures have been completed as part of an ongoing quality assurance program. For example, laminar airflow hoods (LAH) should be cleaned before use, compounding equipment should be inspected and maintained according to manufacturers' recommendations, and temperature control equipment should be monitored for temperature and be equipped with an alarm that sounds when the temperature exceeds predefined limits. All equipment maintenance should be completed on a schedule and documented. Equipment cleaning, maintenance, and use should be recorded in individual equipment logs.

Nonsterile Compounding

All equipment and accessories used in compounding should be thoroughly cleaned after each use. Maintenance should be completed on the schedule recommended by the manufacturer and recorded. Weighing equipment should be certified at least annually. Guidelines for checking torsion balances can be found in pharmacy reference texts such as *Remington's Pharmaceutical Sciences* or the *United States Pharmacopeia* and the *National Formulary*.

Sterile Compounding

Sterile parenteral solutions must be kept free of living microorganisms, particulate matter, and pyrogens. This can be done by following several practices to maintain the sterile compounding area. See Chapter 16 in the *ASHP Manual for Pharmacy Technicians,* 4th edition for complete USP standards and information.

A sterile compounding area should be cleaned daily and segregated from normal pharmacy operations, patient specimens, nonessential equipment, and other materials that produce particles. Floors should be disinfected daily, and trash should be removed frequently. Stricter standards must be maintained if Risk Level II (batched solutions) or Risk Level III (sterile solutions from nonsterile ingredients) products are prepared in the area.

Laminar Airflow Workbench

The manufacturer's recommendations for proper operation and maintenance of LAFWs should be followed (see Chapter 1, Figure 6 for an illustration of the LAFW). LAFWs should be tested by qualified personnel every 6 months, whenever the hood is moved, or if filter damage is suspected. The LAFW should be cleaned before use; HEPA filters should be inspected every 6 months and have their prefilters changed regularly.

Before use, all interior working surfaces of the LAFW should be cleaned with 70% isopropyl alcohol or other appropriate disinfecting agent and a clean, lint-free cloth. The sidewalls of the hood should be cleaned in an up and down direction, starting at the HEPA and working toward the outer edge of the hood. The walls are generally cleaned before the "floor" of the hood. The hood should be cleaned often throughout the compounding period and when the work surface becomes dirty. LAFWs must be cleaned and disinfected at a minimum frequency of the beginning of each shift, before each batch, not longer than 30 minutes following the previous surface disinfection when ongoing compounding activities are occurring, after spills, and when surface contamination is known or suspected. Some materials are not soluble in alcohol and may initially require the use of water in order to be removed. After the water is applied and wiped off, the surface should be cleaned with alcohol. In addition, Plexiglas sides, found on some types of laminar flow workbenches, should be cleaned with warm, soapy water rather than alcohol because the alcohol will dry out the Plexiglas and cause it to become cloudy and possibly cracked. Spray bottles of alcohol should not be used in the hood, as they do not allow for the physical action of cleaning the hood, they can accidentally damage the HEPA filter, and they do not ensure that alcohol is applied to all areas of the surface to be cleaned. Once applied, alcohol should also be allowed to air dry, as this will increase its effectiveness as a disinfectant.

Cleaning should be done periodically during use when the surface is soiled. Any cleaning procedure should take into consideration what drugs have been mixed in the space. If toxic materials have been used in the LAH, proper protective equipment should be used during cleaning. Cleaning materials should be properly disposed of to protect others from exposure.

Biological Safety Cabinet

One of the most important pieces of equipment for handling hazardous drugs safely is the Biological Safety Cabinet (BSC). BSCs must be operated continuously, 24 hours per day, and they should be inspected and certified by qualified personnel every 6 months. Follow the manufacturer's recommendations for proper operation and maintenance, particularly replacement of HEPA filters.

Clean and disinfect the BSC regularly. Clean the work surface, back, and sidewalls with water or a cleaner recommended by the cabinet manufacturer. Do not use aerosol cleaners; they could damage the HEPA filters and cabinet, and could allow contaminants to escape.

Automated Compounders

Equipment used inside the LAFW must be cleaned daily according to the manufacturer's instructions. These systems also require routine maintenance and calibration to ensure accurate compounding measurements.

Repackaging Equipment

Equipment used in repackaging may provide a medium for cross-contamination. Like equipment used in compounding, it should be cleaned after each use.

? Pop Quiz!

How many refills may be ordered for a prescription for alprazolam?

Medication Errors

Pharmacists are responsible for the safe and appropriate use of medications in all pharmacy practice settings. As part of the multidisciplinary health care team, the pharmacist's role is to establish patient-specific drug therapy regimens designed to achieve predefined therapeutic outcomes without subjecting the patient to undue harm. As pharmacists become more involved in patient-specific care, technicians are permitted to perform tasks that were previously restricted to pharmacists. As their responsibilities expand, the role of technicians in ensuring medication safety also increases. As a result, they need to be aware of potential causes of medication errors and the significance of their role in preventing those errors.

According to the *ASHP Guidelines on Preventing Medication Errors in Hospitals,* medication errors can be categorized into 11 types, including:

- prescribing errors
- omission errors
- wrong time errors
- unauthorized drug errors
- improper dose errors
- wrong dosage form errors
- wrong drug preparation errors
- wrong administration technique errors
- deteriorated drug errors
- monitoring errors
- compliance errors

Note that the specific category to which an error belongs is not always obvious, because of the complex nature of the medication use process. Errors can occur because of multiple factors, and therefore may fit into several categories.

Causes of Medication Errors

- Calculation errors—These include misplaced decimal points and using wrong conversions.
- Abbreviations—The Joint Commission has developed a list of dangerous abbreviations and dose designations that should not be used. Technicians should know the list of abbreviations approved by their facility.
- High-alert medications—Because of their high risk of causing serious harm to patients when given in error. Errors with drugs designated as high alert do not necessarily occur more frequently than others. According to the ISMP, the following medications are examples of high alert medications:
  - heparin
  - narcotics and opiates (eg, morphine, hydromorphone, oxycodone)
  - potassium chloride injection
  - insulin
  - chemotherapeutic agents (eg, methotrexate, vincristine, doxorubicin)
  - neuromuscular blocking agents (eg, vecuronium, cisatracurium, succinylcholine)

  A complete list of high-alert medications and drug classes can be found on the ISMP Web site.
- Illegible handwriting

Look-Alike and Sound-Alike Drug Names

Many case reports deal with medication errors caused by confusion surrounding drug names. Hundreds of drug names either sound or look like other trade or generic drug names. The USP provides an easy to use search tool called USP's Drug Error Finder on their Web site. See the appendix "Confused Drug Names" in the *ASHP Manual for Pharmacy Technicians,* 4th edition.

Deteriorated Medications

Because expired medications and improperly stored medications may have lost their potency and thus effectiveness, technicians should take steps to keep these medications out of the dispensing stock. In many cases, it is the technician's responsibility to rotate stock. Technicians should be familiar with the pharmacy's regular system for checking for expired medications. Although checking expiration dates is sometimes viewed as a tedious job, it is important because it reduces the risk of making deteriorated drug errors.

Prevention of Medication Errors

It is impossible to eliminate all potential for error. People are not perfect, and even the most conscientious and knowledgeable staff members can make mistakes. There are several systems and methods that help to prevent medication errors, including failure mode and effects analysis, systems designed to prevent medication errors, legal requirements, policies and procedures, multiple check systems, standardized order forms, education and training, and computerization and automation.

Failure Mode and Effects Analysis

Sometimes the systems that people work within present numerous opportunities for errors. **Failure mode and effects analysis (FMEA)**, also called failure mode effect and criticality analysis (FMECA), is a systematic evaluation of a process or system used to predict the opportunity for and severity of errors at various steps in the process. FMEA focuses on finding flaws within a system that create opportunities for individuals to make errors. It evaluates the "how" and "why" of an error instead of the "who."

Pharmacy Laws

Pharmacy laws are designed to protect the public by ensuring that a knowledgeable individual double-checks the results of the prescribing process and oversees the use of medications.

Policies and Procedures

Policies and procedures formally establish a system to prevent medication errors. Therefore, technicians should be familiar with the workplace's policies and procedures.

Multiple Check Systems

Another system designed to prevent medication errors is a multiple check system. This can include the pharmacist reviewing a physician order, a pharmacy technician preparing a medication for the pharmacist to check, a nurse inspecting the dose from the pharmacy, and a patient asking questions and examining the medication before taking it. A multiple check system is especially important with potentially lethal drugs such as cancer chemotherapeutic agents.

Education and Training

Education and training are important in reducing medication errors. Training can include pharmacy calculations, compounding techniques, pharmacy abbreviations, preparation of IV medications, and computer operation skills. Health care personnel should be familiar with the classes of medications, their generic and trade names, and their forms and doses. The Joint Commission requires organizations to prove their personnel are competent.

Computerization and Automation

The proper use of computerization and automation are effective ways to prevent medication errors. Many health care facilities use bar coding, automated dispensing cabinets (ADC), and robots to reduce medication errors. The technology reduces the number of health care personnel who handle the medications, which can in turn reduce the risk for human error.

What to Do When an Error Occurs

Whatever the circumstances surrounding an actual medication error, the pharmacy technician has a responsibility to inform the pharmacist about any known details. Pharmacists usually investigate the error and the severity of the consequences and gather the details before contacting the physician. The pharmacy technician must follow his or her institution's policy and procedures for the reporting of medication errors.

Liability

Technicians and pharmacists need to be informed about how to prevent medication errors. In addition to the institution or company liability, they may be held personally accountable for a medication error involving injury to a patient.

Identifying Trends

One of the purposes of medication error review is to look for medication errors that occur frequently or involve high-risk medications. The reviewers look for trends among medication error reports and evaluate the systems involved in the errors. Many quality assurance committees focus on the pharmacy's processes (eg, staff orientation and education) instead of on individual staff members, because most medication errors are due to poor drug distribution systems, miscommunication, faulty pharmaceutical packaging, labeling, nomenclature, and lack of information rather than any one person. Education is important to prevent other associates from making similar mistakes.

Self-Assessment Questions

1. What topics do policies and procedures generally cover?
   a. steps to follow when making an IV solution
   b. how the pharmacy should respond in an emergency
   c. staffing levels for the pharmacy
   d. how drug distribution is done
   e. all of the above
2. Quality control programs make sure that processes are working the way they are expected to, whereas quality improvement programs strive to make processes work better than before.
   a. True
   b. False
3. If a patient is out of refills but needs the medication, which of the following is (are) true for the pharmacist?
   a. can dispense an emergency supply if the physician cannot be contacted
   b. cannot dispense an emergency supply without violating the law
   c. can call the physician to obtain refills for the patient
   d. can refill the prescription without calling the physician if it is obvious that the medication is supposed to be continued
   e. both a and c
4. Which of the following medications are exempt from the Poison Prevention Packaging Act?
   a. oral contraceptives
   b. nitroglycerin
   c. medications packaged for patient use by the manufacturer
   d. all of the above
   e. no drugs are exempt from this important safety legislation
5. Schedule I drugs have a high abuse potential and are only rarely used medically.
   a. True
   b. False
6. Benzodiazepines like diazepam, lorazepam, and triazolam are schedule _______ drugs.
   a. II
   b. III
   c. IV
   d. V
7. What does OBRA 90 require?
   a. that pharmacists make the offer to counsel
   b. that the offer to counsel be made in writing
   c. that the pharmacist include a number of elements in education, including what to do if a dose is missed
   d. that there be a minimum of two pharmacists on duty at all times so that one is available to do counseling
   e. that someone provide counseling, but that person can be a pharmacist or a technician—whoever is free at the time
8. The Health Insurance Portability and Accountability Act of 1996 (HIPAA) strengthened patient privacy protection for health information.
   a. True
   b. False
9. Record retention rules vary by state, but the minimum amount of time most records should be retained is 7 years.
   a. True
   b. False
10. Laws that govern pharmacy technicians are the same in all 50 states.
    a. True
    b. False
11. ________ is responsible for registering or licensing pharmacy technicians.
    a. PTCB
    b. ASHP
    c. NABP
    d. State Boards of Pharmacy

Self-Assessment Questions

12. Nonverbal communication includes body language,
    a. appearance, and behavior
    b. physical distance, and physical contact
    c. how the message is spoken
    d. a and b
    e. all of the above
13. AMP is the average price
    a. paid by the wholesaler
    b. paid by the pharmacy
    c. paid by the manufacturer
    d. paid by the self-pay patient
14. The plan whereby a drug company offers certain free drugs to low-income patients who lack prescription drug coverage is
    a. indemnity insurance
    b. Medicare Part D
    c. patient assistance program
    d. WAC
15. PBMs
    a. are organizations that administer pharmacy benefits for private insurance companies
    b. are organizations that administer pharmacy benefits for third party insurance providers
    c. are organizations that administer pharmacy benefits for the federal government
    d. are organizations that administer pharmacy benefits for private or third party payers.
16. Medicare is
    a. a medical and long-term care program funded by federal and state governments
    b. the federal health program for the elderly, disabled, and others with ESRD and ALS
    c. the federal health program for low-income Americans
17. Medicare Part D plans all subscribe to the same formulary with the same costs and benefits to all subscribers.
    a. True
    b. False
18. ICD-9 codes used in claim submissions are used to designate
    a. beneficiaries
    b. drug name, strength, and manufacturer
    c. place of service
    d. diagnosis
19. How should laminar airflow hoods be cleaned?
    a. with water and disinfected with 70% isopropyl alcohol
    b. from the dirtiest area to the cleanest
    c. always the same way regardless of what was last prepared in the hood
    d. both a and b
    e. none of the above
20. What should routine maintenance of the sterile compounding area include?
    a. LAH pre-filter should be changed monthly
    b. floor should be cleaned daily
    c. trash should be emptied frequently
    d. HEPA filter should be inspected every 6 months
    e. all of the above
21. When cleaning a laminar flow hood the technician should
    a. work from the outer edge toward the HEPA, then move to the floor
    b. start with the floor, then the walls from the outer edge toward the HEPA
    c. work from the HEPA toward the outer edge, then the floor
    d. start with the floor, then move to the walls starting at the HEPA toward the outer edge
    e. it all works as long as it gets done
22. Biological safety cabinets should
    a. be left running 24 hours a day
    b. be turned on only when in use and closed when not in use
    c. replace all LAFWs
    d. be cleaned with aerosol cleaners to assure adequate coverage

Self-Assessment Questions

23. According to the ISMP, insulin is a high alert drug.
    a. True
    b. False
24. Failure Mode and Effective Analysis (FMEA) is a systematic approach evaluating
    a. who is causing errors in the drug-use process
    b. what process should be fixed to eliminate errors in the drug-use process
    c. how and why an error was made in the drug-use process.
    d. standardized training of pharmacy technicians to minimize errors in the drug-use process
25. Because pharmacists have the responsibility for the final check of all products, the pharmacy technician is free of all liability.
    a. True
    b. False

Self-Assessment Answers

1. e
2. a
3. e
4. d
5. b
6. c
7. c
8. a
9. b
10. b
11. d
12. e
13. c
14. c
15. d
16. b
17. b
18. d
19. a
20. e
21. c
22. a
23. a
24. c
25. b

Chapter 4

Pharmacy Calculations Review

Learning Outcomes

After completing this chapter, the technician should be able to:

- Define Arabic numbers and Roman numerals.
- Perform basic mathematical functions involving fractions.
- Convert easily among fractions, decimals, percentages, and mixed numbers.
- Work with various measurement systems, including metric and household, and convert measurements in one system to equivalent measurements in other systems.
- Perform temperature conversions between centigrade and Fahrenheit.
- Perform time conversions between 12-hour time and 24-hour time.
- Perform body surface area (BSA) and ideal body weight (IBW) calculations.
- Perform pharmacy calculations involving ratio/proportion.
- Perform dosage calculations including daily doses, and days supply calculations.
- Perform IV flow rate calculations.
- Perform simple statistical calculations.

This chapter reviews the fundamentals of calculations and how those calculations are applied in pharmacy. For additional review and practice problems, see Chapter 14, Pharmacy Calculation, in *Manual for Pharmacy Technicians*, fourth edition.

Kinds of Numbers

Arabic numbers is the system of notation that is preferred in pharmacy practice. This is the system we are most familiar with, consisting of the numbers 0, 1, 2, 3, 4, 5, 6, 7, 8, and 9. From these numbers, fractions and decimal numbers are written.

Roman numerals consist of a numbering system using letters to represent numbers. Roman numerals are used to designate numbers and are often used in prescription writing to designate quantities to be dispensed or the number of a unit of medication the patient is to take. Roman numerals are used in prescription writing because they are more difficult to alter in the case of controlled substances. The following rules apply to the Roman numbering system:

- When a Roman numeral of equal or lesser value is placed after one of equal or greater value, the value of the numerals is added.
- A numeral cannot be repeated more than three times.
- When a Roman numeral of lesser value is placed before a numeral of greater value, the value of the

first numeral is subtracted from the numeral of greater value.

Roman Numeral	Numeric Value
ss	1/2
I or i	1
V or v	5
X or x	10
L or l	50
C or c	100

Examples: IX = 10 – 1 = 9
iii = 3
XL = 50 – 10 = 40

Review of Basic Mathematical Functions Involving Fractions

All fractions must be converted to a common denominator when adding and subtracting. When multiplying and dividing, however, this conversion is not necessary. When working with fractions, the answer should be expressed as the smallest reduced fraction (ie, if the answer is 6/8, it should be reduced to 3/4).

Addition

The following steps are necessary to add these fractions: 3/4 + 7/8 + 1/4

1. Convert all fractions to common denominators:
   3/4 × 2/2 = 6/8
   1/4 × 2/2 = 2/8
2. Add: 6/8 + 7/8 + 2/8 = 15/8
3. Reduce to the smallest fraction:
   15/8 = 1 7/8

Subtraction

The following steps are necessary to subtract these fractions: 7/8 – 1/4

1. Convert the fractions to common denominators:
   1/4 × 2/2 = 2/8
2. Subtract: 7/8 – 2/8 = 5/8

Multiplication

The following steps are necessary to multiply these fractions: 1/6 × 2/3

When multiplying and dividing fractions, it is not necessary to convert to common denominators.

1. Multiply the numerators: 1 × 2 = 2
2. Multiply the denominators: 6 × 3 = 18
3. Express the answer as a fraction: 2/18
4. Reduce the fraction: 2/18 = 1/9

Division

The following steps are necessary to divide these fractions: 1/2 ÷ 1/4

Once again, it is not necessary to convert to common denominators.

To divide two fractions, the first fraction must be multiplied by the inverse (or reciprocal) of the second fraction.

1. Invert the second fraction: 1/4 becomes 4/1.
2. Multiply: 1/2 × 4/1 = 4/2
3. Reduce to lowest fraction: 4/2 = 2

Converting Fractions to Decimal Numbers

To convert a fraction to a decimal number, the numerator is simply divided by the denominator.

For example, 1/2 = 1 divided by 2 = 0.5

Converting Mixed Numbers to Decimal Numbers

The process of converting mixed numbers to decimal numbers involves the following two steps:

1. Write the mixed number as a fraction.
   Method: Multiply the whole number and the denominator of the fraction. Add the product (result) to the numerator of the fraction, keeping the same denominator.
   Example: 2 ¾ = [(2 × 4) + 3]/4 = 2 times 4 plus 3 over 4 = 11/4
2. Divide the numerator by the denominator.
   Example: 11/4 = 11 divided by 4 = 2.75

An alternate method involves the following three steps:

1. Separate the whole number and the fraction.
   Example: 2 3/4 = 2 and 3/4
2. Convert the fraction to its decimal counterpart.
   Example: 3/4 = 3 divided by 4 = 0.75
3. Add the whole number to the decimal fraction.
   Example: 2 plus 0.75 = 2.75

Converting Decimal Numbers to Mixed Numbers or Fractions

The process of converting decimal numbers to mixed numbers involves the following two steps:

1. Write the decimal number over 1, dividing it by 1. (Remember that dividing any number by 1 does not change the number.)
   Example: 3.5 = 3.5/1
2. Move the decimal point in both the numerator and denominator an equal number of places to the right. The number of places the decimal point needs to be moved is determined by the number of digits following the decimal point in the numerator.
   Example: Because there is only one digit following the decimal point in 3.5, move the decimal point one place to the right in both the numerator and the denominator: 3.5/1 = 35/10.
   The number will remain the same as long as the same steps are taken with the numerator and the denominator. Remember that the decimal point of a whole number always follows the last digit.
3. Simplify the fraction.
   Example: 35/10 = 7/2 = 3 ½

Medication errors can occur when decimals are used incorrectly or misinterpreted. Sloppy handwriting, stray pen marks, and poor quality faxed copies can lead to misinterpretation. Decimal point errors can lead to medication underdoses or overdoses.

Rules Governing Use of Decimals

1. Decimals should only be used when absolutely necessary. For example, five milligrams should be written as 5 mg, not 5.0 mg; the decimal point and **trailing zero** are not necessary. Use of a trailing zero in this example could be misinterpreted as 50 mg.
2. Only zeros serving as place holders should be included after the decimal. For example, if you wish to write seven and five hundredths, it should be written as 7.05 with no zeros following the last significant digit (in this case, the 5).
3. A decimal point should not appear without a number before it. If you wish to write one-half milligram, it should be written as 0.5 mg, not .5 mg. This is referred to as proper use of a **leading zero.** Failure to use a leading zero in this example could lead someone to mistakenly read the number as 5 mg rather than 0.5 mg.

Percentages

Percentage (%) means "by the hundred" or "in a hundred." Percents are just fractions, but fractions with a set denominator. The denominator is always one hundred (100).

Example: "50%" means "50 in a hundred" or "50/100" or "1/2"

Converting Percentages to Fractions

To convert a percentage to a fraction, one would write the number preceding the percent sign over 100 and simplify the resulting fraction.

Example: 25% = 25/100 = 1/4

Converting Fractions to Percentages

Percentage means "by the hundred" or "in a hundred." Percents are fractions with a denominator of 100.

To convert a fraction to a percentage, one must take the following steps to convert the fraction to one in which the denominator is a hundred. This is easiest when the fraction is in the form of a decimal.

1. Write the fraction in its decimal form.
   Example: 3/4 = 3 divided by 4 = 0.75
2. Write the decimal over 1.
   Example: 0.75/1
3. To obtain 100 as the denominator, move the decimal point two places to the right. To avoid changing the value, move the decimal point two places to the right in the numerator as well.
   Example: 0.75/1 = 75/100
4. Because we already know that "out of a hundred" or "divided by a hundred" is the same as percent, we can write 75/100 as 75%.

Concentration Expressed as a Percentage

Percent weight-in-weight (w/w) is the grams of a drug in 100 grams of the product.

Percent weight-in-volume (w/v) is the grams of a drug in 100 milliliters (ml) of the product.

Percent volume-in-volume (v/v) is the milliliters of drug in 100 ml of the product.

These concentration percentages will be discussed in detail a little later in this chapter.

Ratio and Proportion

A ratio shows the relationship between two items. For example, when calculating a dose, a ratio can be used to show the number of milligrams in the dose required per one kilogram of patient weight, which is written as mg/kg and read as "milligrams per kilogram." Two ratios with the same units can be combined to create a **proportion**, or a statement of equality between two ratios.

Example:

Ratio: diphenhydramine 12.5 mg/5 mL means there are 12.5 mg of diphenhydramine in every 5 mL of cough syrup. If we wanted to determine how many mg of diphenhydramine were in 10 mL of cough syrup, we could set up a proportion.

5 g of dextrose in 100 mL of water (this solution is often abbreviated "D5W").

Therefore: 5 g of dextrose in 100 ml of a D5W solution equals 50 g of dextrose in 1,000 mL of a D5W solution;

or

5 g/100 mL = 50 g/1,000 mL

If three of the variables of a proportion are known, one can easily solve for the fourth variable. For example, if the standard dose of a medication is 4 mg per kg of patient weight, and the patient weighs 70 kg, we can set up a proportion to determine how many mg of the drug are needed for this patient:

Example:

$$\frac{4\,mg}{kg} = \frac{x\,mg}{70\,kg}$$

"*x*" represents the unknown value (in this case, the number of mg of the drug) that you will find when you solve this problem.

Step 1: Cross multiply

$$\frac{4\,mg}{1\,kg} = \frac{x\,mg}{70\,kg}$$

4 mg × 70 kg = 1 kg × x mg

Step 2: Divide both sides of the equation by 1 kg, so that you isolate the unknown "x" on one side of the equation. Then you can solve for x.

$$\frac{4\,mg \times 70\,kg}{1\,kg} = \frac{1\,kg \times x\,mg}{1\,kg}$$

The kg units on the numerator and denominator cancel each other out, and any amount divided by one is equal to that amount.

$$\frac{4\,mg \times 70\,kg}{1\,kg} = \frac{1\,kg \times x\,mg}{1\,kg}$$

Therefore the equation becomes:

4 mg × 70 = x mg

x = 280 mg

Problem Solving by the Ratio and Proportion Method

The ratio and proportion method is an accurate and simple way to solve certain problems. To use this method, the technician should learn how to arrange the terms correctly and must know how to multiply and divide.

There is more than one way to write a proportion. The most common is the following:

Term #1/Term #2 = Term #3/Term #4

This expression is read, "Term #1 is to Term #2 as Term #3 is to Term #4."

By cross multiplying, the proportion can now be written as follows:

(Term #1) × (Term #4) = (Term #2) × (Term #3)

Example 1: How many grams of dextrose are in 10 ml of a solution containing 50 g of dextrose in 100 ml of water (D50W)?

The following steps are necessary to solve this problem:

1. Determine which is the known ratio and which is the unknown ratio. In this example, the known ratio is "50 g of dextrose in 100 ml of solution." The unknown ratio is "*X* g of dextrose in 10 ml of solution."
2. Write the unknown ratio (terms #1 and #2) on the left side of the proportion. Be sure that the unknown term is on the top.
   X g/10 mL = Term #3/Term #4
3. Write the known ratio (terms #3 and #4) on the right side of the proportion. The units of both ratios must be the same—the units in the numerators and the units in the denominators must match. In this case, that means grams in the numerator and milliliters in the denominator. If units of the numerators or the denominators differ, then a conversion to the same units must be completed.
   X g/10 mL = 50 g/100 mL
4. Cross multiply.
   X g × 100 mL = 50 g × 10 mL
5. Divide each side of the equation by the known number on the left side of the equation. This will

leave only the unknown value on the left side of the equation:
X g = 50 g × 10 mL/100 mL

6. Simplify the right side of the equation to solve for X grams:

Answer: X g = 5 g

Example 2: The technician needs to prepare a 500-mg chloramphenicol dose in a syringe. The concentration of chloramphenicol solution is 250 mg/ml. How many milliliters should be drawn up into the syringe?

The following steps are necessary to solve this problem:

1. Determine the known and unknown ratios.
   Known: 1 mL/250 mg
   Unknown: *X* mL/500 mg
2. Write the proportion:
   X mL/500 mg = 1 mL/250 mg
3. Cross multiply:
   X mL × 250 mg = 1 mL × 500 mg
4. Divide:
   X mL = 1 mL × 500 mg/250 mg
5. Simplify:
   X ml = 2 mL

Answer: Draw up 2 mL in the syringe to prepare a 500-mg dose of chloramphenicol.

Units of Measure

Metric System

The metric system is based on the decimal system, in which everything is measured in multiples or fractions of ten.

Standard Measures

The standard measure for length is the *meter,* the standard measure for weight is the *gram,* and the standard measure for volume is the *liter.*

Prefixes

The prefixes below are used to describe multiples or fractions of the standard measures for length, weight, and volume.

Latin prefixes

micro- (mc): 1/1,000,000	= 0.000001
milli- (m): 1/1,000	= 0.001
centi- (c): 1/100	= 0.01
deci- (d): 1/10	= 0.1

Latin prefixes denote fractions.

Greek prefixes

deca- (da):	10
hecto- (h):	100
kilo- (k):	1,000
mega- (M):	1,000,000

Greek prefixes denote multiples.

Prefixes with Standard Measures

Length

The standard measure is the meter (m).

1 kilometer (km)	= 1,000 meters (m)
0.001 kilometer (km)	= 1 meter (m)
1 millimeter (mm)	= 0.001 meter (m)
1,000 millimeters (mm)	= 1 meter (m)
1 centimeter (cm)	= 0.01 meter (m)
100 centimeters (cm)	= 1 meter (m)

Volume

The standard measure is the liter (L).

1 milliliter (mL)	= 0.001 liter (L)
1,000 milliliters (mL)	= 1 liter (L)
1 microliter (mcl)	= 0.000001 liter (L)
1,000,000 microliters (mcl)	= 1 liter (L)
1 deciliter (dl)	= 0.1 liter (L)
10 deciliters (dl)	= 1 liter (L)

Weight

The standard measure is the gram (g).

1 kilogram (kg)	= 1,000 grams (g)
0.001 kilogram (kg)	= 1 gram (g)
1 milligram (mg)	= 0.001 gram (g)
1,000 milligrams (mg)	= 1 gram (g)
1 microgram (mcg)	= 0.000001 gram (g)
1,000,000 micrograms (mcg)	= 1 gram (g)

Oral solid medications are usually expressed in mg or g. Liquid medications are usually expressed in mL or L. When filling medication orders, it is critically important that the technician pays careful attention to the units to prevent medication errors and potential patient harm. If a dose or volume is not available commercially, the correct amount must be compounded or measured. Doing so may require converting between units of the metric system.

Each move of the decimal to the left or to the right represents an increase or decrease. As long as you know the order of prefixes, and the magnitude represented, you can easily convert from one unit to another. The stem of the unit represents the type of measure. If you are converting down the chart, move the decimal to the right and your number will get bigger. If you are converting up the chart, move the decimal to the left and your number will get smaller.

Apothecary System

The apothecary system was originally developed in Greece for use by physicians and pharmacists. This system has historical significance for the profession of pharmacy, but it is being replaced by the metric system. The Joint Commission (TJC) recommends that health care providers avoid using apothecary units because they are largely unfamiliar and often confused with metric units. There has been a decrease in the use of the apothecary system in hospitals, but apothecary units are still used in community pharmacy.

The most common apothecary measures appearing today are the grain and the dram. One grain may represent 65 milligrams (a 5 grain aspirin tablet is equal to 325 mg) or one grain may represent 60 milligrams (a 1 grain thyroid tablet is the same as 60 mg of thyroid). One dram is used to represent 5 mL or 1 teaspoonful. Drams rarely appear on prescriptions but are still used to describe the capacity of prescription vials.

Pop Quiz!

How many milligrams are in a 1¼ grain low-dose aspirin?

Avoirdupois System

The avoirdupois system is a French system of mass that includes ounces and pounds. In the United States, this is the system of mass commonly utilized, in which 1 pound equals 16 ounces. Assume this conversion when performing pharmacy calculations unless otherwise stated.

Household System

The household system is the most commonly used system of measuring liquids in outpatient settings. Prescribers frequently refer to teaspoons or tablespoons when writing prescriptions. It is a good practice to dispense a dosing spoon or oral syringe with both metric and household system units for liquid medications. The patient or the patient's caregiver should be instructed on how to interpret the units of measure on the spoon or oral syringe.

The term *drop* is used commonly; however, caution should be used when working with this measure, especially with potent medications. The volume of a drop depends not only on the nature of the liquid but also on the size, shape, and position of the dropper. To accurately measure small amounts of liquid, use a 1 ml syringe (with milliliter markings) instead of a dropper. Eye drops are an exception to this rule; they are packaged in a manner to deliver a correctly sized droplet.

Equivalencies Between Systems (Table 4-1)

The systems that have been described lack a close relationship among their units. For this reason, the preferred

Table 4-1. Common Conversions

Converting Measures of Length		
Metric		**Household**
2.54 cm	=	1 inch

Converting Measures of Mass		
Metric		**Avoirdupois**
1 kg	=	2.2 pounds (lb)
454 g	=	1 lb
28.4 g (usually rounded to 30 g)	=	1 ounce (oz)

Converting Measures of Volume		
Metric		**Household**
5 mL	=	1 teaspoon (tsp)
15 mL	=	1 tablespoon (T)
30 mL	=	1 fluid ounce (fl oz)
473 mL (usually rounded to 480 mL)	=	1 pint

Converting Within the Household System	
1 cup	8 fluid ounces
2 cups	1 pint
2 pints	1 quart
4 quarts	1 gallon

Converting Temperature	
Metric	**Household System**
degrees Celsius	degrees Fahrenheit

system of measuring is the metric system. The tables of weights and measures below give the approximate equivalencies used in practice.

Using the proportion method, you can convert from household to metric units.

Example:
How many mL in 2.5 teaspoonfuls?

Set up a proportion starting with the conversion you know.

$$\frac{5\,mL}{1\,tsp} = \frac{x\,mL}{2.5\,tsp}$$

To solve for *x,* use the 2-step process of cross multiplying and dividing to isolate *x* so that you can solve for *x:* 5 mL × 2.5 tsp = 1 tsp × *x* mL

$$\frac{5mL \times 2.5tsp}{1\,tsp} = \frac{1\,tsp \times x\,mL}{1\,tsp}$$

$$\frac{5mL \times 2.5tsp}{1\,tsp} = \frac{1\,tsp \times x\,mL}{1\,tsp}$$

5 mL × 2.5 = *x* mL
x = 12.5 mL

Temperature Conversion

Temperature is measured in the number of degrees centigrade (°C), also known as degrees Celsius, or the number of degrees Fahrenheit (°F). The following equation shows the relationship between degrees centigrade and degrees Fahrenheit:

[9(°C)] = [5(°F)] – 160°

Example: Convert 110°F to °C.
[9(°C)] = [5(110°F)] – 160°
°C = (550 – 160)/9
°C = 43.3°

Example: Convert 15°C to °F
[9(15°C)] = [5(°F)] – 160°
(135 + 160)/5 = °F
59° = °F

Time Conversion

It is also important to know how to convert between the 12 hour and 24 hour clock because many institutions refer to medication administration by the 24 hour clock. The 24 hour clock, also known as military time, does not include am or pm to designate hours of the day. Instead, the hours represent the number of hours and minutes since midnight and range from 0–23. It is reported without a colon separating hours and minutes (example: 2130 = 9:30pm)

Example: Convert 4:15 pm to the 24 hour clock.
12 + 4 = 16 hours in the 24 hour clock
Note: 4 PM is 4 hours past 12 noon
4:15 pm = 1615 in the 24 hour clock

It is good practice for individuals to work within the system with which they are most comfortable to minimize error. Most practitioners prefer to work within the metric system because there are fewer conversions to remember. Instead of memorizing all conversions from one system of measure to another, remember key conversions (listed) and then conversions within each system.

Determining Body Surface Area

The square meter surface area (body surface area) is a measurement that is used instead of kilograms to estimate the amount of medication a patient should receive. Body surface area (BSA) takes into account the patient's weight and height. BSA is always expressed in meters squared (m^2) and is frequently used to dose chemotherapy agents. The following equation is used to determine BSA. When using the equation below, units of weight (W) should be kilograms (kg), and height (H) should be centimeters.

For example, a man weighing 150 lbs (68.2 kg) and standing 5'10" (177.8 cm) tall has a BSA of 1.8 m^2.

BSA values are frequently used to calculate doses of chemotherapeutic agents. There are several similar equations that are used, such as the Mosteller formula, which is:

$$BSA\,(m^2) = \sqrt{\frac{[height(cm) \times weight(kg)]}{3600}}$$

Find out which equation is preferred at your institution by asking your pharmacist. Hospital computer systems will calculate the BSA value for you. Because this is a complex equation prone to error when performed manually, it is wise to count on the computer system, but to understand how the calculation is performed.

Example: If the dose of a drug was recommended at 0.75 mg/m^2 and we determined the BSA of our patient to be 0.7m^2, what would the recommended dose be for this patient?

0.75 mg/m^2 = x mg/0.7 m^2

X = 0.3 mg would be the recommended dose for this patient.

Ideal Body Weight

Ideal Body Weight (IBW) is an estimate of how much a patient should weigh based on his or her height and gender. IBW is expressed as kg. The formulas for determining IBW are:

IBW (kg) for males = 50 kg + 2.3 (inches over 5')
IBW (kg) for females = 45.5 kg + 2.3 (inches over 5')

Examples:
Calculate the IBW for a 72-year-old male who is 6'2" tall.

IBW (kg) = 50 kg + 2.3(14)
IBW = 82.2 kg

Calculate the IBW for a 52-year-old female who is 5'9" tall.

IBW (kg) = 45.5 kg + 2.3(9)
IBW = 66.2 kg

Body Mass Index

Body Mass Index (BMI) is a measure of body fat based on height and weight. This value is used to determine if a patient is underweight, of normal weight, overweight, or obese. The BMI is not generally used in medication calculations, but it may be mentioned in the pharmacy and in the literature. BMI is calculated using this formula:

$$BMI\left(\frac{kg}{m^2}\right) = \frac{weight\,(kg)}{[height\,(m)]^2}$$

Dosage Calculations

Basic Principles

1. The technician should always look for what is being asked:
   - Number of doses
   - Total amount of drug
   - Size of a dose

   Given any two of the above, the technician can solve for the third.
2. Number of doses, total amount of drug, and size of dose are related in the following way:
   Number of doses = Total amount of drug / Size of dose
   This proportion can also be rearranged as follows:
   Total amount of drug = (number of doses) × (size of dose)
   or
   Size of dose = Total amount of drug/Number of doses
   Dosage calculations can be based on weight, BSA, or age.

Calculating Dose Based on Weight

Certain medications require patient-specific dosing. Depending on the medication, BSA or weight-based dosing may be employed. For example, pediatric dosing is frequently determined by the weight of the child. If diphenhydramine syrup is dosed 5 mg/kg per day, and the child weighs 43 lbs, how many mg should the child receive in one day?

First, convert all necessary values to the appropriate units.

$$\frac{2.2\,lb}{1\,kg} = \frac{43\,lb}{x\,kg}$$

$$x\,kg = \frac{43}{2.2} = 19.5\,kg$$

Second, set up a proportion with the available information, and solve for x.

$$\frac{5\,mg}{1\,kg} = \frac{x\,mg}{19.5\,kg}$$

$$x\,mg = 5\,mg \times 19.5 = 97.5\,mg$$

Dose (in mg) = [dose per unit of weight (in mg/kg)] × [Weight of patient (in kg)]

Dose/day (in mg/day) = [dose/kg per day (in mg/kg per day)] × [Weight of patient (in kg)]

To find the size of each dose, the technician should divide the total dose per day by the number of doses per day, as illustrated in the following formula:

Size of Dose = Total amount of drug/Number of doses

Calculating Dose Based on BSA

BSA is expressed as meters squared (m^2). To calculate the amount of a dose on the basis of BSA, the technician should simply multiply the BSA in m^2 times the dose per m^2 as provided in the order or other labeling.

Day's Supply

Part of the dispensing process is to ensure that a patient receives a sufficient quantity of the medication to last for the desired duration. To determine the **day's sup-**

ply, evaluate the dosing regimen to determine how much medication per dose, then how many times the dose is given each day, and then for how many days the medication will be given.

Example:
Metoprolol 50 mg po twice daily for 30 days (25 mg tablets available)

1. The dose is 50 mg, which will require 2 of the 25 mg tablets. The dose is given twice daily, which will require 2 tablets × 2 = 4 tablets per day.
2. The medication regimen will last 30 days, so 4 tablets per day × 30 days = 120 tablets.

Calculating the quantity needed of an oral medication is fairly straightforward, but calculating topical products may be a bit more challenging. For eye drops, the drops per mL may vary, depending on the viscosity of the drops.

Example:
Betaxolol ophthalmic solution 2 drops in each eye twice daily for 10 days (5 mL dropper bottle available; assume 1 mL = 20 drops for this ophthalmic solution, which is a common estimate for many ophthalmic solutions)

1. The patient will take 4 drops twice daily for a total of 8 drops per day.
2. The patient will use 8 drops per day for 10 days for a total of 80 drops.
3. Set up a proportion to determine mL needed per day.
   $$\frac{8 \text{ drops per day}}{x\ mL \text{ per day}} = \frac{20 \text{ drops}}{1\ mL}$$
   $20 * x\ ml = 8 * 1\ mL$
   $x = 0.4\ mL$ per day
   The patient is taking the medication for 10 days so 0.4 mL * 10 days = 4 mL total volume needed to fill the prescription.
4. Determine if the available product will provide a sufficient quantity of medication. Because the total volume of the dropper vial is 5 mL and this prescription calls for 4 mL, one unit would be dispensed to fill the prescription. It is acceptable for the patient to receive slightly more volume than the calculated amount in case they have difficulty applying the drops and accidentally miss applying the medication in their eyes.

Concentration and Dilution

Some pharmacy mixtures are created by adding two solids together. When this occurs, the percentage strength is measured in weight in weight (w/w) or grams of drug/100 grams of mixture. This measurement is mainly used when compounding ointments and creams. When mixtures are created by adding two liquids together, the percentage strength is measured in volume in volume (v/v) or mL/100 mL. When mixtures are created by adding a solid to a liquid, the percentage strength is measured in weight/volume (w/v) or grams per 100 mL. (Table 4-2)

Concentration Expressed as a Percentage

The concentration of one substance in another may be expressed as a percentage or a ratio strength.

As stated earlier in this chapter, concentrations expressed as percentages are determined using one of the following formulas:

1. Percent weight-in-weight (w/w) is the grams of a drug in 100 grams of the product.
2. Percent weight-in-volume (w/v) is the grams of a drug in 100 mL of the product.
3. Percent volume-in-volume (v/v) is the milliliters of drug in 100 mL of the product.

Table 4-2. Standard IV Solutions

Solution	Also Known As	Also Written As	Contains
NS	normal saline	0.9% NaCl (sodium chloride)	0.9 g NaCl in 100 mL water
1/2NS	half normal saline	0.45% NaCl	0.45 g NaCl in 100 mL water
1/4NS	quarter normal saline	0.225% NaCL	0.225 g NaCl in 100 mL water
D5W	dextrose 5% in water	5% dextrose in water	5 g dextrose in 100 mL water
D10W	dextrose 10% in water	10% dextrose in water	10 g dextrose in 100 mL water
D5NS	dextrose 5% in normal saline	5% dextrose in 0.9% NaCl	5 g dextrose and 0.9 g NaCl in 100mL water

Example 1:
0.9% sodium chloride (w/v) = 0.9 g of sodium chloride in 100 mL of solution.

Example 2:
5% dextrose in water (w/v) = 5 g of dextrose in 100 mL of solution.

Example 3:
How many grams of dextrose are in 1 L of D5W?

The following steps of the ratio and proportion method are necessary to solve this problem:

Known ratio: D5W means 5 g/100 mL
Unknown ratio: *X* g/1 L

1. Write the proportion:
   X g/1 L = 5 g/100 mL
2. It is not time yet to cross multiply. First, convert the denominator of either term so both are the same. Because we know that 1 L = 1,000 mL, the unlike terms should be converted as follows:
   X g/1,000 mL= 5 g/100 mL
3. Now that the units are both in the same order and the units across from each other are the same, cross multiply:
   X g × 100 mL = 5 g × 1,000 mL
4. Divide:
   X g = 5 g × 1,000 mL/100 mL
5. Simplify:
   X g = 50 g

There are 50 g of dextrose in 1 L of D5W.

Here are a few suggestions for solving concentration and dilution problems:

1. Calculate the number of grams in 100 ml of solution first. That is the "known" side of the ratio.
2. Calculate the number of grams in the volume requested in the problem by setting up a ratio.
3. Check to make sure the units are in the same order in the ratio.
4. Make sure the units that are across from each other in the ratio are the same.
5. After arriving at the answer, convert it to the requested units.

Concentration Expressed as a Ratio Strength

Concentrations of weak solutions are frequently expressed as ratio strength.

Example: Epinephrine is available in three concentrations: 1:1,000 (read "one to one thousand"); 1:10,000; and 1:200.

A concentration of 1:1,000 means there is 1 g of epinephrine in 1,000 mL of solution.

What does a 1:200 concentration of epinephrine mean?

It means 1 g of epinephrine in 200 ml of solution.

What does a 1:10,000 concentration of epinephrine mean?

It means 1 g of epinephrine in 10,000 mL of solution.

The pharmacy technician can use this definition of ratio strength to set up the ratios needed to solve problems.

Example: 500 mL of a 1:2500 solution of potassium permanganate is ordered. How many grams of potassium permanganate will need to be weighed to make the solution?

1 gram/2500 mL = x grams/500 mL
X = 0.2g

Dilutions Madc from Stock Solutions

Stock solutions are concentrated solutions used to prepare various dilutions of the original stock solution. To prepare a solution of a desired concentration, the technician must calculate the quantity of stock solution that must be mixed with diluent to prepare the final product.

Calculating Dilutions

Example 1: A 10% NaCl stock solution is available. The technician needs to prepare 200 mL of a 0.5% NaCl solution. How many milliliters of the stock solution does the technician need to make this preparation? How much more water does the technician need to add to produce the final product?

The following steps are necessary to solve this problem:

1. Calculate how many grams of NaCl are in the requested final product.
   X g NaCl/200 mL soln = 0.5 g NaCl/100 mL soln
   Therefore, 200 mL of 0.5% NaCl solution contains 1 g of NaCl.
2. Calculate how many milliliters of the stock solution will contain the amount calculated in step 1 (ie, 1 g):

Remember, 10% means the solution contains 10 g/100 mL.
X mL/1 g = 100 mL/10 g
X ml = 10 mL
The first part of the answer is 10 ml of stock solution.

3. Calculate how much water is needed to finish preparing the solution.
Keep in mind the following formula:
(final volume) – (stock solution volume) = (volume of water)
Therefore, for the problem "200 mL – 10 mL = 190 mL of water," the second part of the answer is 190 mL of water.

Example 2: The technician has to prepare 500 ml of a 0.45% NaCl solution from a 10% NaCl stock solution. How much stock solution and water are needed?

The following steps are necessary to solve this problem:

1. Calculate how many grams of NaCl are in the requested volume. In other words, 500 ml of a 0.45% NaCl solution contains how much NaCl?
X g NaCl/500 ml = 0.45 g/100 mL
X g × 100 mL = 0.45 g × 500 ml
X g = 0.45 g × 500 ml/100 mL
X g = 2.25 g
2. Calculate how many milliliters of stock solution will contain the amount in step 1 (ie, 2.25 g)?
X ml/2.25 g = 100 ml/10 g
X ml × 10 g = 2.25 g × 100 mL
$$X \text{ ml} = \frac{2.25 \text{ g} \times 100 \text{ mL}}{10 \text{ g}}$$
X ml = 22.5 mL

The technician will need 22.5 ml of stock solution.

3. Calculate how much water the technician will need.
(Final volume) – (stock solution volume) = volume of water 500 mL – 22.5 mL = 477.5 mL water

Answer: The technician will need 22.5 ml of stock solution and 477.5 mL of water to make the final product.

? Pop Quiz!
1 kg = ______ lb.

Alligation Method

At times, the desired concentration of a product is not readily available, but concentrations above and below the desired concentration are available. The **alligation method** will help to determine how many parts of each strength should be mixed together to prepare the desired strength. The easiest way to visualize an alligation is to set up a tic tac toe board, as shown in Figure 4-1.

This column is %.	This column is %.	This column is PARTS.
High concentration →	→	(Desired concentration) – (low concentration) = number of parts of high concentration needed
Low concentration	Desired concentration	
→	→	(High concentration) – (desired concentration) = number of parts of low concentration needed
		Totol parts (add numbers of parts from above)

Figure 4-1. Alligation method. This method helps to determine how many parts of each strength should be mixed together to prepare the desired strength.

%	%	PARTS
45%		15 parts of high concentration
	25%	
10%		20 parts of high concentration
		35 parts total (550 mL)

Figure 14–2. Example of using the alligation method

Example:
You have an order for 550 mL of a 25% solution. You have a 45% solution and a 10% solution available. How many mL of the 45% solution will you need to mix with the 10% solution to prepare the amount of 25% solution that you need? Figure 4-2 shows use of the alligation method to solve this problem.

Therefore the equation will start with that information:

$$\frac{15\,parts}{35\,parts} = \frac{x\,mL}{550\,mL}$$

Using the two-step process of cross multiplying and dividing to isolate x:

$$x\,mL = \frac{15 * 550\,mL}{35} = 235.7 \text{ mL of the 45\% solution}$$

Knowing that the total is 550 mL, you can subtract the amount of the 45% (235.7 mL) from the total to calculate the amount of the 10% solution needed.

$$550\ mL - 235.7\ mL = 314.3\ mL\ of\ 10\%\ solution\ needed$$

It is helpful to double check your work and calculate it both ways.

Remember, if the product does not contain an active ingredient, its concentration is 0%. Similarly, if the product is pure active ingredient, its concentration is 100%.

Another method to solve similar problems uses the equation below:

$$C_1V_1 = C_2V_2$$

C represents concentration, V represents volume, and the subscript numbers represent two different solutions.

Example: You have an order for 5 mL of a 70% ethanol solution. You only have 98% ethanol. How many mL of the 98% solution will you add to sterile water to make 5 mL of the 70% ethanol solution?

$$C_1V_1 = C_2V_2$$

$$98\%_{\text{conc of 98\% soln}}\ X_{\text{volume needed of 98\% soln}} = 70\%_{\text{conc of 70\% soln}}\ 5_{\text{volume desired of 70\% soln}}$$

$$98x = 70 * 5$$

$$x = \frac{70 * 5}{98} = 3.6\,mL$$

So you would add 3.6 mL of the 98% solution with enough sterile water to make 5 mL of the 70% solution.

? Pop Quiz!

In the formula $C_1V_1 = C_2V_2$, what does V_2 represent?

Flow Rate Calculations

IV Flow Rate Calculations

When working in an institutional setting or home care, it is important to know how to perform calculations related to intravenous medications. This includes calculating the rate at which a medication should be infused. Use the math concepts practiced above to find the necessary information.

Flow rates for IV solutions being infused by mechanical means or pumps are measures in milliliters per hour.

Note that all flow rates are whole numbers, both gtts/min and mL/hr.

Examples:

How many mL per minute will a patient receive if a 500 mL solution is infused over 2 hours?

To solve this problem, set up a proportion:

$$\frac{500\,mL}{120\,min} = \frac{x\,mL}{min}$$

$$500 \text{ mL} \times min = 120\ min \times x\ mL$$

$$x\ mL = \frac{500}{120} = 4.2$$

Therefore the rate is 4.2 mL per minute or 4 mL/min.

How many drops per minute will a patient receive if a 250 mL solution is infused over 1 hour and the infusion set delivers 10 drops/mL?

Set up a proportion to determine the mL per minute and then set up a second proportion to determine the number of drops.

$$\frac{250\,mL}{60\,min} = \frac{x\,mL}{1\,min}$$

$$250\ mL \times 1\ min = 60\ min \times x\ mL$$

$$x\ mL = \frac{250}{60} = 4.2\ mL\ per\ minute$$

Now determine how many drops this would be by setting up a second proportion:

$$\frac{10\,drops}{1\,mL} = \frac{x\,drops}{4.2\,mL}$$

x drops = 10 × 4.2 drops per minute

A useful formula for drip(flow) rates is

$$\frac{\text{Volume (mls) (drop rate in gtts/mL)}}{\text{Time (in minutes)}} = \text{gtts/min}$$

Therefore in the above example 250 mL (10 gtts/mL) ÷ 60 min = 42 gtts/min.

What is the infusion rate of an IV fluid being infused by a pump if 1 liter of fluid is to be infused over 24 hours? 1 liter = 1,000 ml so 1,000 ml ÷ 24 hours = 41.67 = 42 ml/hr

Chemotherapy Calculations

Accurate pharmacy calculations are critically important in the oncology setting, where medications administered to patients are extremely potent and can cause patient harm or death if miscalculations occur. A system of checks and rechecks is in place in most institutions that compound chemotherapy to ensure accurate calculations and medication preparation prior to patient administration.

Example: A medication order is received for amifostine 200 mg/m^2 over 3 minutes once daily 15–30 minutes prior to radiation therapy. The patient is a 79-year-old man weighing 157 lbs and standing 6' tall. He has a BSA of 1.9 m^2. What is the dose of amifostine for this patient?

The easiest way to solve this problem is to set up a proportion.

$$\frac{200mg}{m^2} = \frac{xmg}{1.9m^2}$$

$$x\,mg = \frac{200 \times 1.9}{1} = 380\,mg$$

? Pop Quiz!

How many times can a prescription for methylphenidate be refilled?

Statistics

The arithmetic mean is a value that is calculated by dividing the sum of a set of numbers by the total number of number sets. This value is also referred to as an *average*. The following formula is used to determine the average:

$$M = \frac{\Sigma X}{N}$$

Σ = sum

M = mean (average)

X = one value in set of data

N = number of values X in data set

Using the formula, the following steps help one to calculate the arithmetic mean age of five pharmacists whose ages are 25, 28, 33, 47, and 54 years.

1. Calculate the sum of all ages.
2. Divide the sum by total number of pharmacists

$$\frac{25 + 28 + 33 + 47 + 54}{5} = \frac{187}{5} = 37.4 \text{ years}$$

The *median* is a value in an ordered set of values below and above which there are an equal number of values. When an even number of measurements are arranged according to size, the median is defined as the mean of the values of the two measurements that are nearest to the middle. In the previous example, the median age is 33 years.

? Pop Quiz!

If the patient is receiving a 50 mL IVPB over 30 minutes via pump, what is the flow rate?

Specific Gravity

Specific gravity is a number unique to each substance. It is the ratio of the weight of the compound to the weight of the same amount of water. For example, the specific gravity of milk is 1.035 and the specific gravity of ethanol is 0.787. In other words, milk is denser than water and ethanol is less dense than water. Knowing the specific gravity of a substance is helpful when converting between weight and volume. Generally, units do not appear with specific gravity. In pharmacy calculations, specific gravity and density are used interchangeably; therefore we can use the following formula:

$$specific\ gravity = \frac{\text{weight}\,(g)}{\text{volume}\,(mL)}$$

We know that the specific gravity of water is 1, so we can assume that 1 mL of water weighs 1 gram.

Example:
What is the weight of 473 mL of coal tar if the specific gravity is 0.84?

To answer this question, start with the known specific gravity of 0.84, which means 0.84 g/mL, and set up this proportion:

$$\frac{0.04\,g}{1\,mL} = \frac{x\,g}{473\,mL}$$

Solve for x:

$$x\text{ g} = 0.84 \times 473 = 397.3\text{ g}$$

Suggested Reading

From *Manual for Pharmacy Technicians,* 4th ed.:
Pharmacy Calculations: See Chapter 14—Pharmacy Calculations.

Practice Calculations 1

1. Convert IV to its Arabic equivalent:_____
2. Convert III to its Arabic equivalent:_____
3. Write 1/8 as a decimal fraction:_____
4. Write the fraction form of 0.4:_____
5. Express 25% as a fraction:_____
6. Write 0.45 as a percentage:_____
7. Express 2/5 as a percentage:_____
8. Write the fraction form of 0.65:_____
9. Express XXIV in Arabic numbers:_____
10. Express 1 1/4 in decimal form:_____
11. The standard metric system measure for weight is the_____
12. The standard metric system measure for length is the_____
13. The standard metric system measure for volume is the_____
14. 1 m = _____ km
15. 1 mL = _____ L
16. 1 g = _____ kg
17. 1 mg = _____ g
18. 1 mg = _____ mcg
19. 1 mcg = _____ mg
20. 1 L = _____ mL
21. 1 TBS = _____ tsp
22. 1 fl oz = _____ mL
23. 1 tbsp = _____ mL
24. 15 mL = _____ tsp
25. 6 tsp = ________ tbsp
26. 100 mL = _____ L
27. 2 kg = _____ lb
28. 45 mL = __________oz.
29. 7.5 mL = ______ tsp
30. 1 kg = _____ g
31. 1 tsp = _____ mL
32. 5 gr = _____ mg
33. 4 oz. = ________ mL
34. 85 kg = _____ lb
35. 60 mL = _____ fl oz
36. 81 mg = _____ gr
37. 25 mg = _____ g
38. 2 tbsp = _____ tsp
39. 1 fl oz = _____ tbsp
40. 1 gallon = ___________ mL
41. 250 mL = __________ liter
42. 20 mL = _____ tsp
43. 45 mL = _____ tbsp
44. 150 mg = _____ g
45. 1 lb. = ___________g
46. 2.5 L = __________ mL
47. 30 kg = _____ lb
48. 725 mg = _____ g
49. 10 mL = _____ tsp
50. 9 tsp = _____ tbsp
51. 125 mg = __________ mcg
52. 325 mg = _________ grains
53. 45 lb. = _______kg
54. express the ratio 1:2,000 as a percent
55. 4875 mL = ___________ L
56. 4 oz. = _______ g
57. 180 mL = ________ oz.
58. 2.56 g = _________ mcg
59. 250 mcg = ______ mg
60. 8 oz. = _______ ml
61. express 0.05% as a fraction
62. express 0.05% as a ratio
63. express 1 : 10,000 as a percent
64. 0.00345 g = ____________mg
65. 125,000 mg = ___________ kg

Practice Calculations 2

1. A patient is ordered HCTZ 25 mg daily, available are 50 mg scored tablets.
   a. How should the directions on the prescription label read?
   b. How many tablets should be dispensed?
2. A patient is ordered to take 150 mg of Tegretol daily for 30 days. The supply on hand is Carbamazepine 100 mg/5 mL.
   a. How many milliliters should the patient receive per dose?
   b. How many milliliters should be dispensed?
3. You receive an order for Amoxicillin 400 mg BID X 10 days for a child. Your supply is Amoxicillin 400 mg/5 mL.
   a. How should the directions on the prescription label read?
   b. How many milliliters must be dispensed?
4. Metformin is available in 500 mg tablets. The prescription reads: "750 mg Q AM & PM."
   a. How many tablets should the patient take per dose?
   b. How many tablets must be dispensed for a one month supply?
5. Humulin N 100 units/mL 10 ml vials area available. The patient has a prescription that reads "10 units Q AM and 15 units Q PM." How many days will the vial last?
6. Zofran is available in a 100 mL bottle containing 4 mg/5 mL. The patient is taking 10 mg q 12 hours.
   a. How many mL should this patient take per dose?
   b. What is the estimated days supply (EDS) of the 100 mL bottle?
7. Aerobid-M 7 grams (100 inhalations) is prescribed for a patient using two inhalations BID. How many inhalers will the patient need for one month?
8. The prescription reads Digoxin 0.125 mg daily, on hand is Digoxin 125 mcg. How should the directions on the prescription label read?
9. 4% (w/w) = _____
   12% (w/v) = _____
   0.75% (v/v) = _____
10. A patient needs a 350-mg dose of amikacin. How many milliliters does the technician need to draw from a vial containing 100 mg/2 mL of amikacin?
11. A suspension of naladixic acid contains 250 mg/5 ml. The syringe contains 20 ml. How many grams of naladixic acid does the syringe contain?
12. How many milligrams of neomycin are in 250 ml of a 1% neomycin solution?
13. 1/2 NS = _____ g NaCl/_____ mL solution
14. How many grams of pumpkin are in 200 mL of a 25% pumpkin juice suspension?
15. Express 2.5% hydrocortisone cream as a ratio. (Remember that solids, such as creams, are usually expressed as w/w.)
16. The technician has a solution labeled "D10NS."
    a. How many grams of NaCl are in 100 mL of this solution?
    b. How many milliliters of this solution contain 10 g dextrose?
17. A syringe is labeled "inamrinone 5 mg/mL, 10 mL." How many milligrams of inamrinone are in the syringe?
18. Neupogen 480 mcg/1.6 mL, how many milligrams are contained in this vial?
19. Boric acid 1:100 is written on a prescription. This is the same as _____ boric acid in _____ solution.
20. How many grams of epinephrine is necessary to prepare 20 mL of a 1:1,000 epinephrine solution?
21. Calculate the amounts of boric acid and zinc sulfate in grams to fill the following prescription:

Zinc sulfate	0.1%
Boric acid	1:10
Distilled water qs. ad	100 mL

22. Use the following concentrations to solve the problems:

Gentamicin	80 mg/mL

Practice Calculations 2

Magnesium sulfate 50%
Atropine 1:200
a. 160 mg gentamicin = _____ mL
b. 10 mg atropine = _____ mL
c. _____ g magnesium sulfate = 120 mL

23. Use the following concentrations to solve the problems:

Lidocaine 1%
Heparin 10,000 units/mL solution
Folic Acid 5 mg/mL
a. 300 mg Lidocaine = ____________ mL
b. 5000 units Heparin = ______________ mL
c. 0.1 mg Folic Acid = _________ mL

24. Patient has Humalog U-100 KwikPen The prescription reads 5 units Q PM. How many days will one 3 mL pen last the patient?

25. Potassium chloride is supplied in 30 ml vials containing 2 mEq/mL of potassium. An IV order requires 34 mEq of potassium. How many milliliters need to be added?

26. Trileptal 300 mg/5 mL is ordered for a prescription with the directions of 450 mg BID.
    a. How should the directions on the prescription label read?
    b. How many milliliters must be dispensed to provide a 30 day supply?

27. A drug is available as a 1:10,000 solution, how many mcg of drug are in 2 mL?

28. A chemotherapy agent is available in a 5 mg/mL solution. The recommended dose is 25 mg/m^2. What should the dose in milliliters be for a child if the child is 0.24m^2?

29. Amoxicillin is supplied 400 mg/5 mL, based on the recommended dose of 50 mg/kg/day in 3 divided doses, how many milligrams of drug should a 55 lb child receive per dose?

30. How many grams of sodium chloride are in a liter of NS?

Practice Calculations 3

1. The technician needs to prepare 2 L of 0.25% acetic acid irrigation solution. The stock concentration of acetic acid is 25%.
   a. How many milliliters of stock solution are needed?
   b. How many milliliters of sterile water have to be added?
2. A drug order requires 50 ml of a 2% neomycin solution.
   a. How much neomycin concentrate (1 g/2 mL) is needed to fill the order?
   b. How many milliliters of sterile water need to be added to the concentrate before dispensing the drug?
3. a. Calculate the amount of atropine stock solution (concentration 0.5%) needed to compound the following prescription:
   Atropine sulfate 1:1,000
   Sterile water qs ad 300 mL
   b. How much sterile water has to be added to complete the order?
4. How many tablets have to be dispensed for the following prescription?
   Obecalp ii tablets tid for 14 days
5. How many 2-tsp doses can a patient take from a bottle containing 4 fl oz?
6. A patient is receiving a total daily dose of 1 g of acyclovir. How many milligrams of acyclovir is he receiving per dose if he takes the drug five times a day?
7. The recommended dose of erythromycin to treat an ear infection is 50 mg/kg per day given q6h. Answer the following questions regarding this drug:
   a. If a child weighs 15 kg, how much erythromycin should he receive per day?
   b. How much drug will he receive per dose?
8. The dose of prednisone for replacement therapy is 2 mg/m^2 per dose. The drug is administered twice daily. What is the daily prednisone dose for a 1.2-m^2 person?
9. An aminophylline drip is running at 1 mg/kg per hour in a 12-kg child. How much aminophylline is the child receiving per day?
10. A child with an opiate overdose needs naloxone. The recommended starting dose is 5–10 mcg/kg. The doctor writes for "0.3 mg naloxone stat." Answer the following questions on the basis of the child's weight of 35 kg:
    a. What range of doses, in mcg, could be used to start therapy in this child?
    b. On the basis of the answer to "a," does 0.3 mg sound like a reasonable dose?
11. An IV fluid containing NS is running at 125 mL/h.
    a. How much fluid is the patient receiving per day?
    b. How many 1 L bags will be needed per day?
12. A patient has two IVs running: an aminophylline drip at 22 mL/h and saline at 40 ml/h. How much fluid is the patient receiving per day from his IVs?
13. a. You have a liter of 1% Bronkospaz solution. How many grams of Bronkospaz are in the solution?
    b. If the solution of Bronkospaz you made in "a" runs at 40 ml/h, how much Bronkospaz is the patient receiving per day?
    c. If a 50-kg patient should receive up to 1 mg/kg/hr, will the dose in "b" be excessive?
14. If a patient is receiving an IV solution at 25gtt/min, using tubing that delivers 10gtts/mL, how long would one liter of D_5W last?
15. A patient is to receive 250 mL of IV fluid over 2 hours using a 15 gtt set. What would the flow rate be in gtt/min?
16. Medication is ordered at 4 mg/kg daily per IV over 1 hour. The patient weighs 195 lb. The drug is available in a 250 mg/2 mL vial.
    a. How many ml of drug is needed?
17. An IV solution is ordered requiring 250 mL of Drug AX 15%. The stock of Drug AX 20% is available.
    a. How many milliliters of concentrate are needed?
    b. How many milliliters of diluent are needed?

Practice Calculations 3

18. You are to prepare 2 oz. of Folic Acid 100 mcg/mL using a stock of Folic Acid 5 mg/ml.
    a. How much Folic Acid, in milliliters, do you need?
    b. How much diluents, in milliliters, do you need?
19. If an IV is running at 100 mL/hr, how many liter bags are needed for 24 hours?
20. How many grams of coal tar must be added to 1 lb. of 10% coal tar to make a 15% ointment?
21. 425 grams of sucrose is added to 500 mL of water with a resulting volume of 850 ml, express the concentration of sucrose as a w/w and a w/v product.
22. Cleocin T 2% is a topical product used for acne. How many grams of clindamycin would be contained in a 2 oz container?
23. A loading dose of an anticonvulsant medication for children is 20 mg/kg and infused at a rate of 0.5 mg/kg per minute, over how many minutes would a dose be administered for a child weighing 50 lb?
24. A physician orders a 5% ophthalmic ointment. How much drug and how much ophthalmic base (in grams) would be needed to prepare a 3 gram tube of ointment?
25. Express tobramycin 40 mg/ml as a w/v percent.

Answers to Practice Calculations 1

1. 4
2. 3
3. 0.125
4. 2/5
5. ¼
6. 45%
7. 40%
8. 65/100 = 13/20
9. 24
10. 1.25
11. gram
12. meter
13. liter
14. 0.001 km
15. 0.001 L
16. 0.001 kg
17. 0.001 g
18. 1,000 mcg
19. 0.01 mg
20. 1,000 mL
21. 3 tsp
22. 29.57 (30) mL
23. 15 mL
24. 3 tsp
25. 2 tbsp
26. 0.1 L
27. 4.4 lb.
28. 1 ½ oz.
29. 1 ½ tsp
30. 1,000 g
31. 5 mL
32. 325 mg
33. 120 mL
34. 187 lb.
35. 2 oz
36. 1 ¼ grain, assuming 65 mg = 1 grain
37. 0.025 g
38. 6 tsp
39. 2 tbsp
40. 3785 mL
41. 0.25 L
42. 4 tsp
43. 2 ½ tbsp
44. 0.15 g
45. 454 g
46. 2500 mL
47. 66 lb
48. 0.725 g
49. 2 tsp
50. 3 tbsp
51. 125,000 mcg
52. 5 grains
53. 20.45 kg
54. 0.05%
55. 4.8 L
56. 120 g
57. 6 oz.
58. 2,560,000 mcg
59. 0.25 mg
60. 240 mL
61. 1/2,000
62. 1:2,000
63. 0.01%
64. 3.45 mg
65. 0.125 kg

Answers to Practice Calculations 2

1. a. Take one-half tablet daily for 30 days.
   b. 15 tablets
2. a. 7.5 mL
   b. 225 mL
3. a. Give one teaspoonful twice a day for 10 days.
   b. 100 mL
4. a. 1 ½ tablets
   b. 90 tablets
5. 40 days
6. a. 12.5 mL per dose
   b. 4 days
7. One inhaler will last 25 days—check with the patient's third party provider, the patient needs two inhalers for 30 days, however most third party coverage will not allow you to dispense that many.
8. Take one tablet daily.
9. 4 g/100 g
   12 g/100 mL
   0.75 ml/100 mL
10. 7 mL
11. 1 gram
12. 2,500 mg
13. 0.45 g/100 mL
14. 50 g
15. 2.5 g/100 g = 1g/40 grams or a ratio of 1:40
16. a. 0.9 g
    b. 100 mL
17. 50 mg
18. 0.48 mg
19. 1 g in 100 mL
20. 0.02 g
21. 0.1 g zinc sulfate and 10 g boric acid
22. a. 2 mL
    b. 2 mL
    c. 60 g
23. a. 30 mL
    b. 0.5 mL
    c. 0.02 mL
24. 60 days, however, because the pens are only good for 28 days once they have been used, the patient has only 28 days of usable medication.
25. 17 mL
26. a. Take 1.5 teaspoonful twice a day.
    b. 450 mL
27. 200 mcg
28. 1.2 mL (which is 6 mg)
29. 416.67 mg/dose
30. 9 grams

Answers to Practice Calculations 3

1. a. 20 mL stock solution
   b. 1,980 mL sterile water
2. a. 2 mL stock solution
   b. 48 mL stock solution
3. a. 60 mL stock solution
   b. 240 mL sterile water
4. 84 tablets
5. 12 doses
6. 200 mg per dose
7. a. 750 mg per day
   b. 187.5 mg per dose
8. 4.8 mg per day
9. 288 mg per day
10. a. Acceptable dosage range: 175–350 mcg
    b. Yes, it falls within the accepted calculated range.
11. a. 3,000 ml per day
    b. Three 1 L bags per day
12. 1,488 mL per day
13. a. 1,000 mg/1,000 mL or 1 mg/mL or 1 g/1,000 mL or 1 g/L or 1:1,000
    b. 960 mg/day
    c. No, the dose is lower than would be expected (1,200 mg/day).
14. 400 minutes = 6 hours 40 minutes
15. 31.25 = 31 gtt/min.
16. 2.8 mL
17. a. 187.5 mL concentrate
    b. 62.5 mL diluent
18. a. 1.2 mL Folic Acid
    b. 58.8 mL diluent
19. 3 one liter bags
20. 26.7 g
21. 45.9% w/w and 50% w/v
22. 1.2 g
23. 40 minutes
24. 0.15 g of drug and 2.85 g of base
25. 4%

Chapter 5

Commonly Prescribed Medications

Learning Outcomes

After completing this chapter, the technician will be able to:

- Identify the common drug names for each classification.
- Describe unique characteristics of common drugs as appropriate to the class, such as adverse effects, available dosage forms, and therapeutic uses.
- Describe special dispensing precautions for the major classes of drugs.

This chapter applies to all sections of the PTCB exam, but primarily section I, Assisting the Pharmacist in Serving Patients.

The tables in this chapter should be utilized in assisting you in creating monographs for the drugs listed. You should refer to the current top 200 drug lists to add to this list as appropriate.

Respiratory System

Table 5–1. Agents Used to Treat Asthma and Chronic Obstructive Pulmonary Disease

Generic Name	Brand Name	Common Side Effects
Short-acting bronchodilators		
Albuterol	ProAir HFA	Tremors, nervousness, fast heart rate
	Proventil HFA	
	Ventolin HFA	
Metaproterenol	Alupent	
Levalbuterol	Xopenex HFA	
Long-acting bronchodilators		
Salmeterol	Serevent	Tremors, nervousness, fast heart rate
	Serevent Diskus	

Table 5-1. Agents Used to Treat Asthma and Chronic Obstructive Pulmonary Disease (continued)

Generic Name	Brand Name	Common Side Effects
Formeterol	Formeterol	
Theophylline	Various brands	Nausea, vomiting, fast heart rate, headache, insomnia
Tiotropium	Spiriva	
Inhaled corticosteroids		
Triamcinolone	Azmacort, Nasacort AQ	Thrush, hoarseness
Budesonide	Pulmicort, Rhincocort Aqua	
Fluticasone	Flovent, Flonase, Veramyst, Flovent HFA	
Flunisolide	Aerobid, Aerobid-M	
Beclomethasone	Beconase AQ, Q-Var	
Ciclesonide	Omnaris	Thrush
Mometasone	Nasonex	Thrush
Mast cell stabilizers		
Cromolyn sodium	Intal, Nasalcrom	Headache
Anticholinergics		
Ipratropium	Atrovent HFA	Flushing, dry mouth, constipation, *confusion* confusion
Leukotriene inhibitors		
Zafirlukast	Accolate	Headache, cough, abdominal pain
Montelukast	Singulair	
Zileuton	Zyflo, Zyflo CR	
Combination agents		
Salmeterol/ Fluticasone	Advair, Advair Diskus	
Ipratropium/ Albuterol	Combivent	

Table 5-2. Antihistamines

Generic Name	Brand Name	Availability
First-generation antihistamines		
Chlorpheniramine	Chlor-Trimeton	OTC
Clemastine	Tavist, Tavist Allergy	OTC
Diphenhydramine	Benadryl	OTC
Hydroxyzine	Atarax	Rx
Promethazine	Phenergan	Rx
Second-generation antihistamines		
Cetirizine	Zyrtec	OTC
Loratadine	Claritin	OTC
Levocertirizine	Xyzal	Rx
Third-generation antihistamines		
Desloratadine	Clarinex	Rx
Fexofenadine	Allegra	Rx

Note: OTC = over the counter; Rx = by prescription.

Table 5-3. Miscellaneous Respiratory Medications

Generic Name	Brand Name	Indication
Dextromethorphan	Various OTC	Antitussive
Guaifenesin	Various OTC	Expectorant

Central Nervous System

Table 5-4. Antidepressants

Generic Name	Brand Name	Common Side Effects
Tricyclic antidepressants		
Amitriptyline	Elavil	Sedation, dry mouth, blurred vision, constipation, difficulty urinating
Nortriptyline	Pamelor	"
Imipramine	Tofranil, Tofranil-PM	"
Desipramine	Norpramin	"
Doxepin	Sinequan, Zonalon	"

Table 5–4. (continued)

Generic Name	Brand Name	Common Side Effects
Clomipramine	Anafranil	"
Monoamine oxidase inhibitors (MAOI)		
Phenelzine	Nardil	Postural hypotension or Hypertensive crisis
Tranylcypromine	Parnate	"
Selective serotonin reuptake inhibitors (SSRI)		
Fluoxetine	Prozac	Nausea, diarrhea, anorexia
Paroxetine	Paxil	"
Sertraline	Zoloft	"
Citalopram	Celexa	"
Escitalopram	Lexapro	"
Fluvoxamine	Luvox, Luvox CR	"
Miscellaneous agents		
Nefazodone	Serzone	Same as tricyclics
Trazodone	Desyrel	"
Venlafaxine	Effexor, Effexor-XR	"
Desvenlafaxine	Pristiq	"
Duloxetine	Cymbalta	Black Box suicide warning, nausea, dry mouth, consitpation
Bupropion	Wellbutrin, Wellbutrin-SR, Zyban	Seizures
Mirtazapine	Remeron	Agranulocytosis

Table 5–5. Antipsychotics

Generic Name	Brand Name	Dosage Forms
Conventional antipsychotics		
Low-potency		
Chlorpromazine	Thorazine	Tablets, concentrated liquid, suppositories, injection
Thioridazine	Mellaril	Tablets, suspension
Intermediate-potency		
Perphenazine	Trilafon	Tablets, concentrated liquid

Table 5–5. (continued)

Generic Name	Brand Name	Dosage Forms
Loxapine	Loxitane	Capsules, concentrated liquid
High-potency		
Trifluoperazine	Stelazine	Tablets, concentrated liquid
Fluphenazine	Prolixin	Tablets, deconoate injection, liquid, elixir
Thiothixene	Navane	Capsules
Halperidol	Haldol	Tablets, concentrated liquid, injection, deconoate liquid
Atypical antipsychotics		
Clozapine	Clozaril	Tablets
Olanzepine	Zyprexa	Tablets
Risperidone	Riserdal	Tablets, solution
Quetiapine	Seroquel	Tablets
Ziprasidone	Geodon	Capsules
Aripiprazole	Abilify	Tablets

Table 5–6. Sedatives and Hypnotics

Generic Name	Brand Name	Uses
Benzodiazepines		
Alprazolam	Xanax	Anxiety, sedation
Chlordiazepoxide	Librium	Anxiety
Clorazepate	Tranxene	Anxiety, sedation
Diazepam	Valium	Anxiety, status epilepticus, muscle relaxant
Lorazepam	Ativan	Anxiety, status epilepticus, muscle relaxant
Midazolam	Versed	Sedation in surgical procedures
Oxazepam	Serax	Anxiety
Estazolam	Prosom	Sedation
Flurazepam	Dalmane	Sedation; longest-acting hypnotic
Temazepam	Restoril	Sedation
Triazolam	Halcion	Sedation; shortest-acting hypnotic

Table 5–6. Sedatives and Hypnotics (continued)

Generic Name	Brand Name	Uses
Quazepam	Doral	Sedation
Other agents (nonbenzodiazepines)		
Buspirone	Buspar	Low abuse potential, less sedating than benzodiazepines, used for anxiety
Zolpidem	Ambien, Ambien CR	Sedation
Zaleplon	Sonata	Sedation
Eszopiclone	Lunesta	Sedation
Ramelteon	Rozerem	Sleep maintenance
Secobarbital	Seconal	Sedation
Choral Hydrate	Aquachloral	Procedure sedation

Table 5–7. Anticonvulsants

Generic Name	Brand Name	Seizure Indication
Phenobarbital	Luminal	Tonic-clonic, partial and febrile
Phenytoin	Dilantin	Status epilepticus, tonic-clonic
Fosphenytoin	Cerebyx	Status epilepticus, tonic-clonic
Diazepam	Valium	Status epilepticus
Lorazepam	Ativan	Ativan
Clonazepam	Klonopin	Absence, myoclonic
Valproic acid	Depakene	Absence
Divalproex Na	Depakote	Absence, partial
Ethosuximide	Zarontin	Absence
Carbamazepine	Tegretol, Tegretol-XR	Tonic-clonic, partial
Primidone	Mysoline	Tonic-clonic
Gabapentin	Neurontin	Tonic-clonic, partial
Oxcarbazepine	Trileptal	Partial
Lamotrigine	Lamictal	Partial
Felbamate	Felbatol	Partial
Levetiracetam	Keppra	Adjunctive to partial
Tiagabine	Gabitril	Adjunctive to partial
Zonisamide	Zonegran	Adjunctive to partial

Table 5–7. (continued)

Generic Name	Brand Name	Seizure Indication
Topiramate	Topamax	Adjunctive to tonic-clonic, partial
Pregabalin	Lyrica	Adjunctive therapy, management of fibromyalgia

Table 5–8. Anti-Parkinson Drugs

Generic Name	Brand Name	Drug Action
Levodopa/ carbidopa	Sinemet, Sinemet CR	Increased dopamine in the brain
Tolcapone	Tasmar	Decreased break-down of levodopa
Entacapone	Comtan	Decreased break-down of levodopa
Amantadine	Symmetrel	Mimic or increase the activity of dopamine
Bromocriptine	Parlodel	Mimic or increase the activity of dopamine
Pergolide	Permax	Mimic or increase the activity of dopamine
Selegiline	Eldepryl	Eldepryl
Pramipexole	Mirpex	Stimulates dopamine receptors
Rasagiline	Azilect	MAOI
Ropinirole	ReQuip, ReQuip XL	Stimulates dopamine receptors
Benztropine	Cogentin	Anticholinergic effects
Biperiden	Akineton	Anticholinergic effects
Procyclidine	Kemadrin	Anticholinergic effects
Trihexyphenidyl	Artane	Anticholinergic effects

Table 5–9. Anti-Migraine (Triptans)

Generic Name	Brand Name	Common Side Effects
Almotriptan	Axert	Drowsiness, hot flashes, nausea, vomiting
Eletriptan	Replax	Nausea, drowsiness, dizziness

Table 5–9. (continued)

Generic Name	Brand Name	Common Side Effects
Frovatriptan	Frova	Dizziness, hot/cold sensations
Naratriptan	Amerge	Dizziness, drowsiness
Rizatriptan	Maxalt, Maxalt XLT	Dizziness, drowsiness
Sumatriptan	Imitrex	Dizziness
Zolmitriptan	Zomig	Dizziness, drowsiness

Cardiovascular System

Table 5–10. Antihyperlipidemics

Generic Name	Trade Name	Common Side Effects
Bile acid sequestrants		
Cholestyramine	Questran	Constipation, nausea, gas, abdominal cramping
Colestipol	Colestid	"
Colesevelam	Welchol	"
CoA reductase inhibitors (statins)		
Fluvastatin	Lescol	Headache, GI upset, muscle and joint pain, abnormal liver function tests
Lovastatin	Mevacor	"
Atorvastatin	Lipitor	"
Pravastatin	Pravachol	"
Simvastatin	Zocor	"
Rosuvastatin	Crestor	"
Fibrates		
Gemfibrozil	Lopid	GI symptoms, dizziness, taste disturbances, headache
Fenofibrate	Tricor	"
Fenofibric acid	Trilepix	"
Miscellaneous agents		
Nicotinic acid	Niacin, Niaspan	Flushing, GI symptoms

Table 5–10. (continued)

Generic Name	Trade Name	Common Side Effects
Niacin/lovastatin	Advicor	
Ezetimibe	Zetia	GI symptoms, arthralgia
Ezetimibe/ simvastatin	Vytorin	"
Atorvastin/ amlodipine	Caduet	

Note: GI = gastrointestinal.

Table 5–11. Miscellaneous Antihypertensives

Generic Name	Brand Name	Drug Action
Doxazocin	Cardura	Alpha-1 blocker
Prazocin	Minipress	Alpha-1 blocker
Terazosin	Hytrin	Alpha-1 blocker
Clonidine	Catapres	Alpha-2 agonist
Guanabenz	Wytensin	Alpha-2 agonist
Methyldopa	Aldomet	Alpha-2 agonist
Hydralazine	Apresoline	Direct vasodilator
Minoxidil	Loniten	Direct vasodilator
Aliskiren	Tekturna	Renin inhibitor

Table 5–12. Diuretics

Generic Name	Brand Name	Comments
Thiazide diuretics		
Hydrochlorothiazide (HCTZ)	Hydrodiuril, Microzide	May cause loss of potassium, may alter blood glucose levels
Chlorothiazide	Diuril	"
Indapamide	Lozol	"
Chlorthalidone	Hygroton	"
Metolazone	Zaroxolyn	"
Loop diuretics		
Furosemide	Lasix	More potent than thiazides, causes loss of potassium
Bumetanide	Bumex	"
Torsemide	Demadex	"
Ethacrynic acid	Edecrin	"

Table 5–12. Diuretics (continued)

Generic Name	Brand Name	Comments
Potassium-sparing diuretics		
Spironolactone	Aldactone	Potassium supplements usually not needed, often used in combination with thiazides to increase potency
Triamterene	Dyrenium	"
Combination agents		
Triamterene/HCTZ	Dyazide, Maxzide	Diuretics
Spironolactone/ HCTZ	Aldactazide	Diuretics
Amiloride/HCTZ	Moduretic	Diuretics
Losartan/HCTZ	Hyzaar	ARB/diuretic
Lisinopril/HCTZ	Zestoretic	ACE-I/diuretic
Bisoprolol/HCTZ	Zebeta	Beta-blocker/diuretic
Valsartan/HCTZ	Diovan HCT	ARB/diuretic
Olmesartan/HCTZ	Benicar HCT	ARB/diuretic

Note: ARB = angiotesin II receptor blocker; ACE-I = angiotensin-converting enzyme inhibitor.

Table 5–13. Beta-Blockers, Ace Inhibitors, and Arbs

Generic Name	Brand Name	Comments
Beta-blockers		Note - *olol* ending Contraindicated in patients with asthma or diabetes
Atenolol	Tenormin	"
Metoprolol	Lopressor, Toprol-XL	"
Nadolol	Corgard	"
Propranolol	Inderal, Inderal LA	"
Timolol	Blocadren, Timoptic	"
Carteolol	Cartrol	"
Bisoprolol	Zebeta	"
Pindolol	Visken	"
Sotalol	Betapace	"
Acebutolol	Sectral	"
Carvedilol	Coreg	"

Table 5–13. (continued)

Generic Name	Brand Name	Comments
Labetolol	Normodyne, Trandate	"
Nebivolol	Bystolic	"
Betaxolol	Kerlone	"
ACE inhibitors		Note: *pril* ending, may cause dry cough, may not require potassium supplements; patients with diabetes may use for kidney protective qualities
Benazepril	Lotensin	"
Enalapril	Vasotec	"
Fosinopril	Monopril	"
Lisinopril	Prinivil, Zestril	"
Quinapril	Accupril	"
Ramipril	Altace	"
Tramdolapril	Mavik	"
Perindopril	Aceon	"
Moexipril	Univasc	"
Angiotensin II receptor blockers (ARBs)		Note: *artan* ending, does not cause dry cough; effects similar to ACE-Is
Valsartan	Diovan	"
Irbesartan	Avapro	"
Candesartan	Atacand	"
Telmisartan	Micardis	"
Eprosartan	Teveten	"
Olmesartan	Benicar	"

Table 5–14. Calcium Channel Blockers

Generic Name	Brand Name	Comments
Dihydropyridines		Note: *dipine* ending
Amlodipine	Norvasc	
Nifedipine	Procardia XL, Adalat CC	Headache, flushing, and gum overgrowth are side effects
Felodipine	Plendil	
Isradipine	DynaCirc	

Table 5–14. (continued)

Generic Name	Brand Name	Comments
Nicardipine	Cardene SR	
Nimodipine	Nimotop	
Nondihydropyridines		
Diltiazem	Cardizem (SR, CD), Tiazac, Dilacor XR	Nausea, headache are common
Verapamil	Calan SR, Verelan, Isoptin SR, Covera HS	

Table 5–15. Antiarrhythmics

Generic Name	Brand Name	Class
Lidocaine	Xylocaine	Class I, Group IB
Tocainide	Tonocard	Class I, Group IB
Mexilitine	Mexitil	Class I, Group IB
Quinidine	Quinaglute, Quinidex	Class I, Group IA
Procainamide	Procan, Procan SR, Pronestyl	Class I, Group IA
Disopyramide	Norpace, Norpace CR	Class I, Group IA
Flecainide	Tambocor	Class I, Group IC
Acebutolol	Sectrol	Class II
Esmolol	Brevibloc	Class II
Propranolol	Inderal	Class II
Propafenone	Rythmol	Class III
Amiodarone	Cordarone, Pacerone	Class III
Sotalol	Betapace	Class III
Dofetilide	Tikosyn	Class III
Ibutilide	Covert	Class III
Diltiazem	Cardizem	Class IV
Verapamil	Isoptin, Calan	Class IV

Table 5–16. Miscellaneous Cardiac Drugs

Generic Name	Brand Name	Indication
Nitroglycerin	Various	Angina
Isosorbide Dinitrate	Dilatrate, Isordil, Sorbitrate	Angina
Isosorbide Mononitrate	Imdur, Ismo, Monoket	Angina
Digoxin	Lanoxin	Heart failure

Table 5–17. Anticoagulants/Antiplatelets/Thrombolytics

Generic Name	Brand Name	Class
Warfarin	Coumadin	Coumarin/ anticoagulant
Heparin		Unfractionated heparin
Enoxaparin	Lovenox	Low molecular weight heparin
Dalteparin	Fragmin	Low molecular weight heparin
Tinzaparin	Innohep	Low molecular weight heparin
Ivalirudin	Angiomax	anticoagulant
Fondaparinux	Arixta	anticoagulant
Lepirudin	Refludan	anticoagulant
Abciximab	ReoPro	antiplatlet
ASA	various	antiplatlet
Clopidogrel	Plavix	antiplatlet
Prasugrel	Effient	antiplatlet
Ticlopidine	Ticlid	antiplatlet
Tirobiban	Aggrastat	Antiplatlet
Alteplase	Activase	thrombolytic
Reteplase	Retevase	thrombolytic
Tenecteplase	TNKase	thrombolytic

Gastrointestinal System

Table 5–18. Drugs Used to Treat Gastro-Esophageal Reflux Disease

Generic Name	Brand Name	Dosage Forms
Proton pump inhibitors		
Omeprazole	Prilosec	Capsule
Pantoprazole	Protonix	Tablet, injection
Lansoprazole	Prevacid	Capsule, suspension
Rabeprazole	Aciphex	Tablet
Esomeprazole	Nexium	Capsule
Histamine-2 antagonists		
Cimetidine	Tagamet	Tablet, oral liquid,

Table 5–18. Drugs Used to Treat Gastro-Esophageal Reflux Disease (continued)

Generic Name	Brand Name	Dosage Forms
Ranitidine	Zantac	Capsule, effervescent granules, syrup, tablet, injection
Famotidine	Pepcid	Capsule, tablet, powder for oral suspension, injection
Nizatidine	Axid	Capsule, tablet
Gastrointestinal stimulants		
Metoclopramide	Reglan	Tablet, oral solution, syrup, injection

Musculoskeletal System

Table 5–19. Nonsteroidal Anti-Inflammatory Agents

Generic Name	Brand Name	Comments
Ibuprofen	Motrin, Advil	Note: *profen* ending
Ketoprofen	Orudis	"
Flurbiprofen	Ansaid	"
Diclofenac	Voltaren	
Sulindac	Clinoril	
Ketoralac	Toradol	Indicated for short-term use only
Naproxen	Naprosyn, Naprelan	
Mecloxicam	Mobic	
Piroxicam	Feldene	
Nabumetone	Relafen	
Fenoprofen	Nalfon	
Oxaprozin	Daypro	
Indomethacin	Indocin	Used to treat gout
Tolmetin	Tolectin	
Cox-2 Inhibitors		Note: *coxib*
Celecoxib	Celebrex	

Table 5–20. Analgesics

Generic Name	Brand Name	Dosage Forms
Major opiates		
Morphine	Various MS Contin	Tablet, sustained-release tablet, injection, oral solution, suppository
Hydromorphone	Dilaudid	Tablet, oral liquid, injection, suppository
Meperidine	Demerol	Tablet, syrup, injection
Fentanyl	Sublimaze, Duragesic, Actiq, Fentanyl Oralet	Injection, transdermal patch, lozenge
Minor opiates		
Codeine		Tablet, oral solution, injection
Oxycodone	Percolone, Oxycontin, Roxicodone	Tablet, capsule, sustained-release tablet, oral liquid
Propoxyphene	Darvon	Capsule, tablet
Nalbuphine	Nubain	Injection
Butorphanol	Stadol	Injection, nasal spray
Dezocine	Dalgan	Injection
Non-opiates		
Acetaminophen	Tylenol	Caplet, capsule, tablet, chewable tablet, drops, elixir, oral liquid, suppository, suspension, drops
Tramadol	Ultram	Tablet
Combination		
Acetaminophen/codeine	Various, Tylenol #3, Tylenol #4, Tylenol/Cod. Elixir	Tablets, elixir
Hydrocodone/acetaminophen	Various, Lorcet, Vicodin	Tablets, elixir
Oxycodone/acetaminophen	Various, Percocet, Roxicet, Tylox	Tablets, concentrated oral solution, elixir

Table 5–21. Neuromuscular Blocking Agents

Generic Name	Brand Name
Succinylcholine	Anectine, Quelicin
Tubocurarine	
Mivacurium	Mivacron
Rocuronium	Zemuron
Pancuronium	Pavulon
Atracurium	Tracrium
Vecuronium	Norcuron
Doxacurium	Nuromax

Table 5–22. Skeletal Muscle Relaxants

Generic Name	Trade Name	Dosage Forms
Carisoprodol	Soma, Rela	Tablet
Chlorzoxazone	Parafon Forte	Caplet, tablet
Cyclobenzaprine	Flexeril	Tablet
Metaxolone	Skelaxin	Tablet
Methocarbamol	Robaxin	Tablet, injection
Orphenadrine	Norflex	Tablet, sustained-release tablet, injection
Lioresal	Baclofen	Tablet
Tizanidine	Zanaflex	Tablet

Endocrine System

Table 5–23. Insulin

Insulin Type	Onset of Action	Duration of Action
Rapid-acting		
Humalog, Lispro	5–15 min.	3–4 hr.
Novolog, Aspart	10–20 min	3–5 hr
Apidra, glulisine	10–15 min	3–5 hr
Short-acting		
Regular	30–60 min.	6–10 hr
Intermediate-acting		
NPH	1 –2 hr	16–24 hr

Table 5–23. (continued)

Insulin Type	Onset of Action	Duration of Action
Long-acting		
Levemir, detemir	0.8–2 hr	no significant peak
Lantus, glargine	1.1 hr	relatively flat

Table 5–24. Oral Hypoglycemics

Generic Name	Brand Name	Comments
Sulfonylureas - first generation		
Chlorpropamide	Diabinese	Long-acting agent
Sulfonylureas-second generation		May be used as monotherapy or in combinations
Glyburide	Micronase, Diabeta, Glynase	
Glipizide	Glucotrol, Glucotrol XL	
Glimepiride	Amaryl	
Meglitinides (secretogogues)		May be used as monotherapy or with Metformin
Nateglinide	Starlix	
Biguanides		
Metformin	Glucophage Glucophage XR	Once daily formulation helps with GI discomfort
Thiazolidinediones (Glitazones)		Monitor liver enzymes
Rosiglitazone	Avandia	
Pioglitazone	Actos	
Alpha-glucosidase inhibitors		
Acarbose	Precose	Take with meal
Miglitol	Glyset	
Dipeptidyl Peptidase Inhibitors		
Sitagliptin	Januvia	
Miscellaneous		
Exenatide	Byetta	Injection, before meals

Table 5–24. Oral Hypoglycemics (continued)

Generic Name	Brand Name	Comments
Combination agents		
Glyburide/ metformin	Glucovance	
Glipizide/ metformin	Metoglip	
Rosiglitazone/ metformin	Avandamet	

Infectious Diseases

Table 5–25. Antibiotics

Aminoglycosides		
Generic Name	**Brand Name**	**Route of Administration**
Gentamicin	Garamycin	Injection
Tobramycin	Nebcin	Injection

Cephalosporins		
Generic Name	**Brand Name**	**Route of Administration**
First-generation agents		
Cefadroxil	Duricef	Oral
Cephalexin	Keflex	Oral
Cefazolin	Ancef, Kefzol	IV, IM
Second-generation agents		
Cefaclor	Ceclor	Oral
Loracarbef	Lorabid	Oral
Cefoxitin	Mefoxin	IV
Cefuroxime	Zinacef, Ceftin	IV, IM, oral
Cefprozil	Cefzil	Oral
Cefpodoxime	Vantin	Oral
Third-generation agents		
Ceftriaxone	Rocephin	IM, IV
Cefdinir	Omnicef	Oral
Cefotaxime	Claforan	IV, IM
Cefditoren	Spectracef	Oral

Table 5–25. (continued)

Cephalosporins		
Generic Name	**Brand Name**	**Route of Administration**
Fourth-generation agent		
Cefepime	Maxipime	Injection

Fluoroquinolones		
Generic Name	**Brand Name**	**Route of Administration**
Ciprofloxacin	Cipro	Oral, IV
Levofloxacin	Levaquin	Oral, IV
Lomefloxacin	Maxaquin	Oral
Moxifloxacin	Avelox	Oral, IV
Ofloxacin	Floxin	Oral

Macrolides Fluoroquinolones		
Generic Name	**Brand Name**	**Route of Administration**
Azithromycin	Zithromax	Oral, IV
Clarithromycin	Biaxin	Oral
Dirithromycin	Dynabac	Oral
Erythromycin	Various	Oral, IV, topical

Penicillins		
Generic Name	**Brand Name**	**Route of Administration**
Penicillin G	Bicillin, Bicillin LA	IM, IV
Penicillin VK	Various	Oral
Penicillinase-Resistant		
Cloxacillin	Dynapen, Pathocil	Oral, Injection
Nafcillin	Unipen	Oral, IV
Broad-spectrum		
Amoxicillin	Various	Oral
Amoxicillin/ clavulanate	Augmentin	Oral
Ampicillin	Principen, Unasyn	Oral, Injection

Note: IV = intravenous; IM = intramuscular.

Table 5–26. HIV Agents

Generic Name	Brand Name	Comments
Reverse transcriptase inhibitors		
Nucleoside reverse transcriptase inhibitors (NRTI)		
Zidovudine	Retrovir	May cause severe anemia, lactic acidosis, and enlarged liver
Didanosine	Videx	Take on empty stomach; may cause lactic acidosis and enlarged liver
Zalcitabine	Hivid	May cause peripheral neuropathies, lactic acidosis, and enlarged liver
Stavudine	Zerit	May cause lactic acidosis and enlarged liver
Lamivudine	Epivir	May cause lactic acidosis and enlarged liver
Abacavir	Ziagen	May cause lactic acidosis and enlarged liver
Abacavir/ lamivudine	Epzicom	May cause lactic acidosis and enlarged liver
Zidovudine/ lamivudine	Combivir	May cause lactic acidosis and enlarged liver
Zidovudine/ lamivudine/ abacavir	Trizivir	May cause lactic acidosis and enlarged liver
Nucleotide reverse transcriptase inhibitors		
Tenofovir	Viread	May cause lactic acidosis and enlarged liver
Non-nucleoside reverse transcriptase inhibitors (NNRTI)		
Nevirapine	Viramune	Severe hepatotoxicity
Efavirenz	Sustiva	Dizziness, headaches, rash, nausea, headaches, elevated hepatic function
Delavirdine	Rescriptor	Dizziness, headaches, rash, nausea, headaches, elevated hepatic function
Efavirine	Sustiva	Headaches, dizziness, insomnia, fatigue, rash, nightmares
Protease inhibitors (PIs)		
Indinavir	Crixivan	Take on empty stomach
Ritonavir	Norvir	Take with food; refrigerate capsules, not solution
Nelfinavir	Viracept	Diarrhea and hyperglycemia are common side effects
Amprenavir	Agenerase	Large quantities of propylene glycol in solution may cause toxicities
Atazanavir	Reyataz	Headaches, diarrhea, nausea, rash
Darunavir	Prezista	Headaches, diarrhea, nausea, rash
Lopinavir/ritonavir	Kaletra	Headaches, diarrhea, nausea, rash
Tipranavir	Aptivus	Headaches, diarrhea, nausea, rash
Fusion Inhibitors		
Enfuvirtide	Fusion	Insomnia, depression, peripheral neuropathy, decreased appetite
CCR5 Antagonists		
Maraviroc	Selzentry	Cough, upper resp, tract infections rash, musculoskeletal symptoms
Integrase Inhibitor		
Raltegravir	Isentress	Nausea, headache, diarrhea, pyrexia

Table 5–27. Chemotherapeutic Agents

Generic Names	Brand Names	Primary Antineoplastic Indications
Alkylating agents		
Busulfan	Myleran	Chromic myelogenous leukemia
Carboplatin	Paraplatin	Ovarian cancer, lung cancer, bladder cancer, breast cancer
Carmustine	BiCNU	Brain tumors, multiple myeloma, melanoma, lung cancer, colon cancer
Chlorambucil	Leukeran	Chronic lymphocytic leukemia, Hodgkin and non-Hodgkin lymphoma, breast cancer, ovarian cancer, testicular cancer

Table 5–27. Chemotherapeutic Agents (continued)

Generic Names	Brand Names	Primary Antineoplastic Indications
Cisplatin	Platinol, Platinol AQ	Head, neck, breast, testicular, bladder cervical, esophageal, and ovarian cancer
Cyclophosphamide	Cytoxan, Neosar	Hodgkin and non-Hodgkin lymphoma, several types of leukemia, neuroblastoma, retinoblastoma
Dacarbazine	DTIC-Dome	Malignant melanoma, Hodgkin disease, soft-tissue sarcomas, fibrosarcomas, islet cell carcinoma of the pancreas, neuroblastoma, thyroid cancer
Ifosfamide	Ifex	Lung cancer, Hodgkin and non-Hodgkin lymphoma, breast, ovarian, and testicular cancers, pancreatic, and gastric carcinoma
Lomustine	CeeNU	Brain tumors, Hodgkin and non-Hodgkin lymphoma, melanoma, renal carcinoma, lung cancer, colon cancer
Mechlorethamine	Mustargen Hydrochloride	Hodgkin and non-Hodgkin lymphoma, epithelial ovarian carcinoma, neuroblastoma, breast cancer
Melphalan	Alkeran	Epithelial ovarian carcinoma, neuroblastoma, breast cancer
Streptozocin	Zanosar	Metastatic islet cell cancer of the pancreas, Hodgkin disease
Antimetabolites		
Cladribine	Leustatin	Hairy cell leukemia, chronic lymphocytic leukemia, non-Hodgkin lymphomas, progressive multiple sclerosis
Cytarabine	Cutosar-U, DepoCyt	Leukemia, lymphoma, meningeal leukemia, meningeal lymphoma
Floxuridine	FUDR	Gastrointestinal adenocarcinoma metastatic to the liver
Fludarabine	Fludara	Chronic lymphocytic leukemia
Fluorouracil	Adrucil	Stomach, colon, rectum, breast, and pancreas cancer
Gemcitabine	Gemzar	Pancreatic cancer, non-small cell lung cancer
Mercaptopurine	Purinethol	Acute leukemias
Methotrexate	Folex PFS	Trophoblastic neoplasms; leukemias, breast, head, neck, stomach, esophagus, testicular, and lung cancers; osteosarcoma
Hormones		
Diethystilbestrol	Stilphosteral	Metastatic prostatic carcinoma and postmenopausal inoperable, progressing breast cancer
Estramustine	Emcyt	Prostatic carcinoma
Flutamide	Eulexin	Metastatic prostatic carcinoma
Letrozole	Femara	Advanced postmeno-pausal breast cancer
Leuprolide	Lupron, Lupron Depot, Lupron Depot-3 Month, Lupron Depot-4 Month, Lupron Depot-Ped	Advanced prostatic cancer, endometriosis central precocious puberty
Medroxyproges-terone	Curretab, Cycrin, Depo-Provera, Provera	Endometrial cancer
Megestrol Acetate	Megace	Breast and endometrial carcinoma
Tamoxifen	Nolvadex	Breast cancer

Table 5–27. (continued)

Generic Names	Brand Names	Primary Antineoplastic Indications
Antibiotics		
Bleomycin	Blenoxane	Squamous cell carcinoma, melanoma, sarcomas, testicular carcinoma, Hodgkin and non-Hodgkin lymphoma
Dactinomycin	Cosmegen	Testicular tumors, melanoma, choriocarcinoma, Wilm tumor, neuroblastoma retinoblastoma, rhabdomyosarcoma, uterine sarcomas, Kaposi sarcoma
Daunorubicin	Cerubidine, DaunoXome	Leukemias, lymphoma, Kaposi sarcoma
Doxorubicin	Adriamycin PFS, Adriamycin RDF, Rubex, Doxil	Leukemias, lymphomas, multiple myeloma; osseous and non-osseous sarcomas; mesotheliomas; germ cell tumors of the ovary or testes; carcinomas of the head, neck, thyroid, and lung; Wilm tumor; breast, stomach, pancreas, liver, ovary, bladder, prostate, and uterine cancer; neuroblastoma
Idarubicin	Idamycin	Acute myeloid leukemia, acute lymphocytic leukemia in children
Mitomycin	Mutamycin	Adenocarcinoma of the stomach or pancreas, bladder cancer, colorectal cancer
Mitoxantrone	Novantrone	Acute nonlymphocytic leukemia, various other leukemias, lymphoma, breast cancer
Mitotic inhibitors		
Docetaxel	Taxotere	Breast cancer, non-small cell lung cancer; under investigation for treatment of gastric, neck, and ovarian cancers, among others
Etoposide	Toposar, VePesid	Lymphomas, leukemias, lung, testicular, bladder, and prostate carcinomas; hepatoma; rhabdomyosarcoma; uterine carcinoma; neuroblastoma; Kaposi sarcoma
Paclitaxel	Paxene, Taxol	Ovarian carcinoma, breast cancer, non-small cell lung cancer, Kaposi sarcoma
Vinblastine	Alkaban-AQ, Velban	Hodgkin and non-Hodgkin lymphoma; testicular, lung, head and neck, breast, and renal carcinomas; Kaposi sarcoma choriocarcinoma
Vincristine	Oncovin, Vincasar PFS	Leukemias, Hodgkin and non-Hodgkin lymphoma, Wilm tumor, neuroblastoma rhabdomyosarcoma
Vinorelbine	Navelbine	Non-small cell lung cancer
Miscellaneous agents		
Asparaginase	Elspar	Acute lymphocytic leukemia, lymphoma
Dacarbazine	DTIC-Dome	Malignant melanoma, Hodgkin disease, soft-tissue sarcomas, fibrosarcomas rhabdomyosarcoma, islet cell carcinoma of the pancreas, medullary carcinoma of the thyroid, neuroblastoma

Table 5–27. Chemotherapeutic Agents (continued)

Generic Names	Brand Names	Primary Antineoplastic Indications
Hydroxyurea	Droxia, Hydrea	Chronic myelogenous leukemia; brain tumors; head and neck tumors; uterine, cervical, and non-small cell lung cancers
Interferon alpha 2a	Roferon-A	Hairy cell leukemia, Kaposi sarcoma, chronic myelogenous leukemia
Interferon alpha 2b	Intron-A	Hairy cell leukemia, malignant melanoma, Kaposi sarcoma, follicular non-Hodgkin lymphoma
Procarbazine	Matulane	Hodgkin and non-Hodgkin lymphoma, brain tumor, bronchogenic carcinoma

Table 5–28. Immunosuppresive Agents

Generic Name	Brand Name	Comments
Cyclosporine	Sandimmune	Hypertension, nephrotoxicity, gingival hyperplasia, nausea, vomiting, diarrhea, hepatoxicity,
Daclizumab	Zenapax	Fever, hypertension, vomiting, wound infection
Mycephenolate	CellCept	Diarrhea, vomiting, leucopenia, neutropenia, infections
Tacrolimus	Prograf	Nephrotoxicity, neurotoxicity, hyperglycemia, nausea, vomiting, infections

Table 5–29. Antivirals

Generic Name	Brand Name	Indications
Acyclovir	Zovirax	Herpes simplex, shingles, genital herpes, chickenpox
Amantidine	Symmetrel	Influenza A
Famciclovir	Famvir	Herpes zoster, genital herpes
Ganciclovir	Cytovene	CMV retinitis, CMV disease
Ribavirin	Virazole	Respiratory Syncytial Virus
Oseltamivir	Tamiflu	Influenza
Valacyclovir	Valtrex	Herpes zoster, genital herpes

Other Conditions

Table 5–30. Agents Used for the Treatment of ADHD

Generic Name	Brand Name	Common Side Effects
Methylphenidate	Concerta, Ritalin, Ritalin SR	Anxiety, insomnia, anorexia
Atomoxetine	Strattera	Headache, nausea, dizziness, vomiting, altered mood, anorexia
Dextroamphetamine/ Amphentamine	Adderall, Adderall XR	Insomnia, talkativeness, anorexia
Lisdexamfetamine	Vyvanse	Anorexia

Table 5–31. Bisphosphonates

Generic Name	Brand Name	Comments
Ibandronate	Boniva	Take at least 60 minutes before first food and beverage, do not lie down for at least 60 minutes after taking, take with 6–8 oz of plain water.
Risedronate	Actonel	Take at least 60 minutes before first food and beverage, do not lie down for at least 60 minutes after taking, take with 6–8 oz of plain water.

Table 5-31. (continued)

Generic Name	Brand Name	Comments
Alendronate	Fosamax	Take at least 30 minutes before first food and beverage, do not lie down for at least 30 minutes after taking, take with 6–8 oz of plain water.

Table 5-32. Phosphodiesterase-5 Enzyme Inhibitors

Generic Name	Brand Name	Common Side Effects
Sildenafil	Viagra	Headache, flushing
Tadalafil	Cialis	Headache, heartburn, flushing, nasal congestion
Vardanafil	Levitra	Headache, flushing, rhinitis, sudden hearing loss

Table 5-33. Agents for the Treatment of Alzheimer Disease

Generic Name	Brand Name	Common Side Effects
Memantine	Namenda	Decreases effect of glutamate
Donepezil	Aricept	Increases concentration of ACH

Topical Medications

Ophthalmic Medications

Table 5-34. Ophthalmic Agents

Generic Name	Brand Name	Dosage Forms
Antibiotic agents		
Gentamicin		Solution, ointment
Tobramycin	Tobrex	Solution, ointment
Na sulfacetamide	Sulf-10	Solution, ointment
Ciprofloxacin	Ciloxan	Solution

Table 5-34. (continued)

Generic Name	Brand Name	Dosage Forms
Ofloxacin	Ocuflox	Solution
Levofloxacin	Quixin	Solution
Norfloxacin	Chibroxin	Solution
Combination agents		
Neomycin/ Polymixin/ Hydrocortisone	Cortisporin	Solution, ointment
Neomycin/Polymixin/ Dexamethasone	Maxitrol	Solution, ointment
Tobramycin/ Dexamethasone	Tobradex	Solution, ointment
Antiviral agents		
Vidarabine	Vira-A	Ointment
Trifluridine	Viroptic	Solution
Ganciclovir	Vitrasert	Implant
Idoxuridine	Herplex	Solution
Antihistamine/decongestant agents		
Lodoxamide	Alomide	
Levocabastine	Livostin	Solution
Ketotifen	Zaditor	Solution
Olopatadine	Patanol	Solution
Emedastine	Emadine	Solution
Azelastine	Optivar	Solution
Antiglaucoma agents		
Beta-blockers		
Betaxolol	Betoptic, Betoptic-S	Solution, suspension
Carteolol	Ocupress	Solution
Levobunolol	Betagan	Solution
Timolol	Timoptic, Timoptic-XE	Solution
Carbonic anhydrase inhibitors		
Dorzolamide	Trusopt	Solution
Brinzolamide	Azopt	Solution
Prostaglandin analog		
Lotanoprost	Xalatan	Solution
Bimatoprost	Lumigan	Solution
Travoprost	Travatan	Solution
Unoprostone	Rescula	Solution

Table 5–34. Ophthalmic Agents (continued)

Generic Name	Brand Name	Dosage Forms
Alpha$_s$ Agonists		
Apraclonidine	Lopidine	Solution
Brimonidine	Alphagan	Solution
Miotics		
Carbachol	Isopto-Carbachol	Solution

Otic Medications

Table 5–35. Common Ingredients in Otic Medications

Ingredient	Indication
Acetic acid	Antibacterial
Aluminum acetate	Antibacterial
Antipyrine	Analgesic
Benzalkonium chloride	Antiseptic
Benzethonium chloride	Antiseptic
Benzocaine	Anesthetic
Boric acid	Drying agent for auditory canal
Hydrocortisone	Corticosteroid
M-cresyl acetate	Antibacterial
Neomycin	Antibacterial
Polymyxin B	Antibacterial

Intranasal Products

Table 5–36. Intranasal Formulations

Generic Name	Brand Name	Onset of Action
Antihistamines		
Azelastine	Astelin	Immediate
Corticosteroids		
Beclomethasone diproprionate	Beconase AQ, Vancenase AQ	Few days to 2 weeks
Budesonide	Rhinocort, Rhinocort AQ	24 hrs
Flunisolide	Nasarel	Few days to 2 weeks
Fluticasone	Flonase	Few days
Mometasone	Nasonex	2 days
Triamcinolone acetonide	Nasacort AQ	12 hrs. to a few days
Mast cell stabilizers		
Cromolyn sodium	Nasalcrom	1–2 weeks
Topical decongestants		
Oxymetazoline	Afrin	Immediate

Dermatological Agents

Table 5–37. Topical Agents

Generic Name	Brand Name	Dosage Forms
Low-potency corticosteroids		
Desonide	DesOwen	Cream, ointment, gel, spray
Hydrocortisone	Various brands	Cream, ointment, gel, spray, solution, lotion
Medium-potency corticosteroids		
Hydrocortisone valerate	Various brands	Cream, ointment
Mometasone	Elocon	Cream, ointment, lotion
High-potency corticosteroids		
Betamethasone diproprionate	Diprosone	Cream, ointment, lotion
Betamethasone	Valerate	Ointment
Desoximetasone	Topicort	Cream, ointment, gel
Fluocinolone	Synalar	Cream, ointment
Fluocinonide	Lidex	Cream, ointment, gel
Halcinonide	Halog	Cream, ointment
Triamcinolone	Various Brands	Cream, ointment, lotion

Table 5–37. (continued)

Generic Name	Brand Name	Dosage Forms
Very high-potency corticosteroids		
Clobetasol	Temovate, Embeline, Cormax	Cream, ointment
Diflorasone	Psorcon-E	Cream, ointment (emollient)
Halobetasol	Ultravate	Cream, ointment
Augmented betamethasone diproprionate	Diprolene	Cream, ointment
Topical antifungals		
Clotrimazole	Lotrimin AF, Mycelex	Cream, lotion, solution
Miconazole	Micatin, Desenex	Cream, powder, spray
Terbinafine	Lamisil AT	Cream
Tolnaftate	Tinactin, Aftate	Cream, solution, powder, aerosol
Ketoconazole	Nizoral	Cream, shampoo
Naftifine	Naftin	Cream, gel
Econazole	Spectazole	Cream

Nutritional Products

Table 5–38. Vitamins

Common Name	Chemical Name	Type (fat-soluble versus water-soluble)
Vitamin A	Retinol	Fat-soluble
Vitamin B_1	Thiamine	Water-soluble
Vitamin B_2	Riboflavin	Water-soluble
Vitamin B_3	Niacin, Nicotinic Acid	Water-soluble
Vitamin B_5	Pantothenic Acid	Water-soluble
Vitamin B_6	Pyridoxine	Water-soluble
Vitamin B_{12}	Cyanocobalamine	Water-soluble
Vitamin C	Ascorbic Acid	Water-soluble
Vitamin D	Ergocalciferol	Fat-soluble
Vitamin E	Tocopherol	Fat-soluble
Vitamin K	Phytonadione	Fat-soluble

Table 5–39. Minerals and Their Functions in the Body

Mineral	Amount Present	Function in Body
Calcium	Major element	Important in bone and tooth formation and in nerve function
Chloride	Major element	Used in the production of hydrochloric acid; closely connected with sodium in body tissues, fluids, and excretions
Chromium	Trace element	A cofactor for insulin
Copper	Trace element	Important for hemoglobin
Fluoride	Trace element	Associated with tooth enamel
Iodine	Trace element	Linked with thyroid function
Iron	Trace element	Important part of the hemoglobin molecule and required in many enzymes
Magnesium	Major element	Second most abundant mineral found in the body; important in body enzymes and in nerve and muscle function
Manganese	Trace element	Needed for growth as well as for various enzymes
Phosphorous	Major element	Important in metabolism and acid-base regulation
Potassium	Major element	Primary mineral found inside cells; important in cellular metabolism and in nerve and muscle function
Selenium	Trace element	Important in cellular metabolism
Sodium	Major element	Important in growth and in muscle function
Sulfur	Major element	Important for many proteins and heparin
Zinc	Trace element	Important for growth and for insulin utilization

Reference:

Saunders Nursing Drug Handbook 2010, Saunders Elsevier, St Louis, Missouri

Suggested Reading

Basic and Clinical Pharmacology. 6th ed. Norwalk, CT: Appleton & Lange; 1995.

Facts and Comparisons. St. Louis, MO: Facts and Comparisons, Inc.

Merck Manual of Diagnosis and Therapy. 16th ed., Rahway, NJ: Merck Research Laboratories; 1992.

USPDI, Volume I, Drug Information for the Health Care Professional. Rockville, MD: United States Pharmacopeia Convention, Inc.;

USPDI, Volume II, Advice for the Patient. Rockville, MD: United States Pharmacopeia Convention, Inc.

Self-Assessment Questions

1. Which drug belongs to the class of calcium channel blockers?
   a. Lidocaine
   b. Calcium carbonate
   c. Nicardipine
   d. Loperidine
   e. Meperidine
2. Which of the following is *not* an opiate analgesic?
   a. Ibuprofen
   b. Hydrocodone
   c. Morphine
   d. Codeine
   e. Hydromorphone
3. Which of the following may be used as antineoplastic agents?
   a. Docetaxel
   b. Doxorubicin
   c. Medroxyprogesterone
   d. Gemcitabine
   e. All of the above
4. Which of the following is *not* a trace element?
   a. Iron
   b. Potassium
   c. Selenium
   d. Chromium
   e. Copper
5. The brand name for cefoxitin is:
   a. Ancef
   b. Rocephin
   c. Fortaz
   d. Mefoxin
   e. Cefizox
6. Which of the following is a diuretic?
   a. Hydroxyzine
   b. Hydrochlorothiazide
   c. Hydroxyurea
   d. Hydrocortisone
   e. Hydrochloric acid
7. Which of the following is *not* used to treat diabetes?
   a. Insulin
   b. Glyburide
   c. Metformin
   d. Metolazone
   e. Pioglitazone
8. Which of the following is the brand name for meperidine?
   a. Demerol
   b. Lasix
   c. Lanoxin
   d. Vicodin
   e. Dilaudid
9. Which of the following is Vitamin B_1?
   a. Folic acid
   b. Riboflavin
   c. Thiamine
   d. Ascorbic acid
   e. Nicotinic acid
10. Which antihistamine is available without a prescription?
    a. Loratidine
    b. Diphenhydramine
    c. Chlorpheniramine
    d. Clemastine
    e. All of the above
11. Which class of drugs used for hypertension ends in "pril"?
    a. ACE Inhibitors
    b. β blockers
    c. Calcium Channel Blockers
    d. Angiotensin II Receptor Blockers
12. Which class of drugs used to treat hypertension ends in "artan"?
    a. ACE Inhibitors
    b. β blockers
    c. Calcium Channel Blockers
    d. Angiotensin II Receptor Blockers
13. Bisphosphonates must be taken
    a. with breakfast
    b. 30–60 minutes (depending on which one is prescribed) before the first food or drink in the morning
    c. after the evening meal
    d. at bedtime

Self-Assessment Questions

14. Viagra is to sildenafil as Levitra is to
    a. tadelafil
    b. donepezil
    c. fluoroluricil
    d. vardanafil
15. Tamiflu is used for
    a. herpes simplex
    b. respiratory syncytial virus
    c. CMV retinitis
    d. influenza
16. Lantus and Levemir have
    a. a peak activity in 16–24 hours
    b. a duration of 6–10 hours
    c. onset of action in less than 60 minutes
    d. have no significant peak
17. Midazolam is used for
    a. treatment of anxiety
    b. sedation before surgical procedures
    c. a hypnotic
    d. for sleep maintenance.
18. Vicodin is a brand name for
    a. oxycodone
    b. hydrocodone
    c. hydrocodone/acetaminophen
    d. hydrocodone/aspirin
19. Which drug listed below is used to treat ADHD?
    a. Tiazac
    b. Arixta
    c. Celebrex
    d. Byetta
    e. Concerta
20. Which drug listed below is NOT a penicillin?
    a. amoxicillin
    b. Augmentin
    c. Biaxin
    d. Unasyn
21. The brand name for atorvastatin is
    a. Crestor
    b. Mevacor
    c. Lipitor
    d. Zocor
22. The drugs known as "triptans" are used to treat
    a. migraines
    b. glaucoma
    c. Parkinson disease
    d. seizures
23. Amantadine is an antiviral used to treat
    a. influenza and glaucoma
    b. influenza and Parkinson disease
    c. influenza and ADHD
    d. influenza and Alzheimer
24. Which drug listed below is NOT a benzodiazepine?
    a. Halcion
    b. Valium
    c. Xanax
    d. Serax
    e. Luensta
25. Cymbalta is used to treat depression and
    a. seizures
    b. glaucoma
    c. insomnia
    d. HIV
26. Guiafenesin is
    a. an antihistamine
    b. an antitussive
    c. an expectorant
    d. a decongestant
27. Which drug listed below is a short-acting bronchodilator?
    a. albuterol
    b. tiotropium
    c. salmeterol
    d. beclamethasone
28. The brand name of pregabalin is
    a. Geodon
    b. Abilify
    c. Keppra
    d. Lyrica
29. Which drug listed below is an anticoagulant?
    a. Activase
    b. Ticlid
    c. Plavix
    d. Coumadin

Self-Assessment Questions

30. Which is the generic name for Nexium?
    a. omeprazole
    b. rabeprazole
    c. esomeprazole
    d. famotidine
31. What is the generic name for Levaquin
    a. levofloxacin
    b. lomefloxacin
    c. moxifloxacin
    d. dirithromycin
32. Vitamin C is
    a. water-soluble
    b. fat-soluble
33. What is the generic name for Singulair?
    a. cetirizine
    b. loratadine
    c. montelukast
    d. zafirlukast
34. Vytorin is used to treat
    a. CHF
    b. hyperlipidemia
    c. angina
    d. insomnia
35. Januvia is used to treat
    a. hyperlipidemia
    b. diabetes
    c. angina
    d. migraines
36. The brand name for desvenlafaxine is
    a. Fluririn
    b. Aciphex
    c. Pritiq
    d. Luenesta
37. The generic name for Skelaxin is
    a. methyphenidate
    b. metaxolone
    c. carisprodol
    d. nizatidine
38. A common side effect of ACE inhibitors is
    a. constipation
    b. gingival enlargement
    c. dry cough
    d. nausea and vomiting
39. Which drug listed below is NOT an SSRI?
    a. Prozac
    b. Lexapro
    c. Celexa
    d. Effexor
40. The generic name for Abilify is
    a. phenelzine
    b. olanzepine
    c. ziprasidone
    d. aripiprazole

Self-Assessment Answers

1. c
2. a
3. e
4. b
5. d
6. b
7. d
8. a
9. c
10. e
11. a
12. d
13. b
14. d
15. d
16. d
17. b
18. c
19. e
20. c
21. c
22. a
23. b
24. e
25. a
26. c
27. a
28. d
29. d
30. c
31. a
32. a
33. c
34. b
35. b
36. c
37. b
38. d
39. d
40. d

Chapter 6

How to Take a Test

Learning Outcomes

After completing this chapter, the technician will be able to:

- Discuss basic study and review skills for objective tests.
- List basic strategies for taking objective tests.
- Define common trouble areas in taking objective tests and describe how to manage these difficulties.
- Recognize test anxiety and define common relaxation techniques.

Revised from the original text written by Nancy F. Fjortoft and Kristin Lange.

You are not alone if you face upcoming examinations with dread and anxiety. Most people do. But exams serve a purpose. They are intended to test your knowledge, not your patience and endurance. Tests are helpful to others who are attempting to determine your understanding and knowledge of specific areas. Tests also help you to understand what areas you are competent in and what areas you need to focus on in terms of your own learning and development.

This chapter reviews preparation tips and test-taking strategies. It concludes with a section on how to deal with the anxiety most of us feel prior to an examination.

Examinations

There are two basic kinds of examinations. The first is the objective examination. Objective examinations include multiple-choice, true/false, and matching questions. Objective examinations are designed to test your ability to recognize, rather than recall, facts and information. The second type is the essay examination. Essay examinations are tests for which respondents give long, written answers. They provide the opportunity for respondents to organize their knowledge, integrate materials, and express themselves. The two kinds of tests require different skill sets. Because your exam will be objective multiple choice, this chapter focuses on techniques to help you perform at your best on this type of examination.

Multiple-Choice Questions

A multiple-choice question normally begins with an incomplete sentence or question, known as a *stem.* The stem is followed by a series of choices for completing the sentence or answering the question, known as *responses.* The responses are usually lettered *a, b, c,* and *d.* Typically, there are four, sometimes five, responses to choose from. You complete the sentence or answer the question by choosing the correct or best response. For example, a typical multiple-choice question will look like this:

(Stem) The capital of Illinois is:

(Responses)

a. Springfield
b. Chicago
c. Rockford
d. St. Louis

Normally, the directions are to pick the one best response. However, the directions vary, so read the directions and the stem carefully. You may be instructed to pick the incorrect option or to pick more than one option. There are also questions that present the stem as a complete statement. Key words to note in the stem are the subject of the question and any qualifiers or adjectives that further define the best answer.

Preparing for Objective Exams

You may be fresh out of the classroom with recent experience in preparing for and taking objective exams, or you might not have taken an exam in quite some time. Whatever the case, it's always useful to review good study skills. This section reviews some basic study and test preparation techniques.

Planning Ahead

The first step in preparing for an exam is to check the date, time, and place of the exam. Mark your calendar and take the time to find the location in advance. You do not want to be late for the exam because you got lost. Estimate how long it will take you to get to the test center. You may even want to do a test drive. Find out where parking is available, or make a trial run on public transportation.

Make sure you understand the scope of the exam. In other words, how long is it and what material will it cover? What materials, if any, can you bring with you? Make sure you understand the purpose and format of the test.

Time Management

Every busy person needs a schedule. But before you can plan your study schedule, you first need a thorough understanding of how you study. Answer these basic questions about yourself:

When is the best time of day for me to study?

How do I best learn?

If you are unsure of the answers to these questions, you may want to monitor yourself for a week. Develop a time chart and follow your activities. Are there any times of the day when you are more productive than others? Think about how you learn as well. What tasks help you learn? Do you learn best by doing or by reading? Some people find reading aloud to be a helpful memorization technique. This kind of self-knowledge will guide you in developing your study schedule. Even though family and work responsibilities may take most of your time, try to use your most productive time of the day for your studies.

Think in small increments of time. Do not postpone studying because you do not have all afternoon to devote to your studies. Plan and organize small learning tasks that can occur in short blocks of time. It is easier to learn when you break your studies into smaller increments. For example, each of these is an increment: review your notes, generate questions from your notes, make a question chart (more on that later) or key word list, and define key words. Don't postpone your studies while you wait for that perfect free day. That free day may not come.

Using Question Charts

One study technique that has been found to be useful in organizing and learning information is a question chart.[1] Question charts help you make connections between information that is new to you and what you already know—an important step in the learning process. For example, if your topic is medication administration, **Table 6-1** gives an example of how to set up your chart.

Make question charts to cover all the main concepts in this review guide. Complete the charts as you read, revising and adding questions as you go, and then use them as study guides.

Defining Terms

Make a separate section in your notes for terms and their definitions. Define each term by a key word or phrase. Review those terms every day, and add terms to your list as you read new material. This is an example of one of the small learning tasks discussed earlier.

Table 6-1. Sample Question Chart

Medication Administration			
Questions	**Intravenous**	**Oral**	**Topical**
What are the available dosage forms?	Solutions, suspensions	Tablets, capsules, solutions, suspensions, powders	Ointments, creams, patches
What are the advantages of this route of administration?	Quick onset of action	Convenience	Limited systemic route of absorption (ointments and creams only)
What are the disadvantages of this route of administration?	No drug recall, pain at injection site	Slower onset of action, taste, palatability	Inconvenience

Group Review

Some people find it helpful to meet with other students to review notes, ask questions, and compare perceptions. This may or may not be helpful to you; it all depends on your personal style. If you do study with others, have an organized agenda so that time is not wasted. Listen and learn from your colleagues, but if you are unsure, check your references. Do not take another person's word for something you are not sure of. Look it up.

Mock Exams

Use your question charts to make up your own exam, or if you are working with a group of colleagues, write questions for each other. This is often a helpful way to prepare for exams. The practice exam included in this book is a good way to test your comprehension of the material.

Final Review

Suppose the test is tomorrow. Spend your final review time reviewing, reciting, and summarizing your notes. When you are reviewing your term list or mastering your notes, make sure that you review from both directions. Begin first with the most difficult material, or reverse the review process by rearranging your notes, reviewing from back to front, and beginning in the middle. Don't get tied to order. If there is anything you are not certain of, now is the time to look it up and learn it. Recite from your summary sheets.

Personal Preparation

Now that you are mentally prepared, prepare yourself physically for your exam. Go to your exam rested. You will not do well on your exam if you are so sleepy that you cannot concentrate on the questions. Eat a good breakfast before your exam. It's hard for the mind to concentrate if the body is demanding attention. Your brain functions better with a supply of energy. Also, it is probably not wise to start a new diet, quit smoking, or begin a new exercise regimen until after you complete the exam. You need to focus your energies on preparing for and taking the exam, not on redesigning your lifestyle.

Prepare emotionally as well. Remember that the purpose of this exam is not to fail you or humiliate you, but to assist you professionally. So relax, be prepared, and concentrate. With preparation and strategy on your side, you will perform at your best.

Taking Objective Exams

You've been preparing for weeks and now the big test date has finally arrived. This section outlines several steps and strategies that are useful in successfully completing an objective test.

Come Prepared

The first step in successfully taking objective tests is to come prepared.

Arrive at the test site 30 to 40 minutes early.

Computerized Testing

Computerized testing poses a unique set of problems. People vary in their level of comfort in dealing with computer programs. If you are not accustomed to working on a computer, it would be wise to complete a practice exam in that format prior to the actual test, if possible. The Pharmacy Technician Certification Board (PTCB) also sells a practice exam on its Web page (www.ptcb.org).

Other programs with computerized standardized tests are available commercially, such as SAT practice programs. These tests may give you practice in computerized testing formats, although the questions will not relate to the Pharmacy Technician Certification Exam.

Computerized tests often employ many of the same types of questions and question formats as paper tests, and you should use most of the same strategies, such as reading both the questions and the answers carefully. One thing that is very different is that your ability to go back and review previous questions is often limited or completely prohibited. It is important for you to try to pace yourself accordingly. Try to make your best answer in the time available to you and move on to the next question. If you are, in fact, able to move backward through the test or parts of it, then you may choose to go back and review your answers. Whether or not this is an option will be made clear in the instructions for the test. If you have a question about looking at already answered questions that is not dealt with in the instructions, you should ask the testing center moderator for additional information. An erasable board will be provided to you to serve as your scratch paper. You should not bring any electronic devices into the testing center, including calculators. You are permitted to use the on-screen calculator or handheld devices provided by the testing center. You will be required to lock all your personal items into a locker during the exam.

Test-Taking Strategies

Some basic strategies are helpful to most people taking objective tests. The first thing every test taker should do is make sure you know how to navigate through the pages of the exam. The PTCB has a tutorial for this that can be accessed from their Web site. You are allowed to mark questions to review later; the exam will prompt you to go back to these questions.

The second step is to use your time wisely. Set yourself a schedule. Using your time wisely is dependent on reviewing the test carefully. The only way to plan your time is to be aware of how many and what types of questions you must answer. You should have an idea of at what time you should be halfway done with the exam. For example, if you have 2 hours for a test, you should be at least halfway through it by the end of the first hour. Remember to leave extra time for particularly tough questions and for review. Work as rapidly as possible with reasonable assurance of accuracy. The PTCB allows 2 hours to complete 90 multiple choice questions.

The third strategy is to read carefully. This includes both the directions and the questions. Sections of the exam may vary, so take the time to read the directions carefully at the beginning of each new section, and keep those directions in mind while answering the questions. Making careless mistakes because you misunderstood the directions is not an effective test-taking strategy! For example, the directions may read, "select the incorrect response," or "mark the two best answers."

Part of reading carefully involves reading the questions as they are, not as you would like them to be. In other words, don't look for answers you have memorized. Answer the question. Many people find it helpful to mark the key words in the stem so they do not forget them or misinterpret them. Also look for and mark the question words. This will help you answer the question as written. Some common question words are *what*, *how*, *when*, and *define*.

A fourth strategy is to leave your assumptions at home. You should not anticipate or assume trick questions. For example, you may know the correct answer is *d,* but you feel you have already answered too many questions with *d.* Take the question at face value and mark the answer you think is correct. Also, do not assume that methods or procedures that you use at work are necessarily the correct ones. "Because that's the way we do it around here" may not be based on fact or best practice.

Going through the test at least two or even three times is another strategy for successful test taking. Go through the test completely the first time and answer all the "easy" questions that you are sure of. While you are doing the first run-through, mark the questions you need to come back to by marking the square in the top left of the page that says "review later." By answering all the easy questions first, you can be assured that you have answered the questions that you know. This strategy also builds confidence. In the stem of one question, you may also find an answer to another question.

On the second run through, answer the questions that you are unsure of by considering all the alternatives and eliminating the options that you know are inappropriate or incorrect. Relate the remaining options to the stem and balance them against each other. Use the information obtained from other questions to help you.

On the third run through, look at the remaining questions. If it is in your best interest to guess, do so. Always guess if your chances of gaining points are greater than your chances of losing points. Use the following strategies for intelligent guessing:

- The most general option is often the correct one because it allows for exceptions. If three of the four options are specific in nature and one is more general, choose the more general option.
- The correct choice is most often a middle value. If the options range in value (for example, from high to low or from big to small), then eliminate the extreme values and choose from the middle values.
- The longest option is often the correct one. If three options are much shorter than the fourth, then choose the longest answer.
- When two options have opposite meanings, then the correct answer is usually one of these.
- Look for grammatical agreement between the stem and the answers. For example, if the stem uses a singular verb tense, then the answer should also be singular. Eliminate the answers that don't produce grammatically correct sentences. Most multiple-choice questions are designed as sentence completions.
- Do not leave questions blank, they will be marked wrong.

Trouble Areas in Objective Exams

A couple of areas are problematic for most people taking objective exams. This section discusses those areas and provides you with some advice on tackling those obstacles.

The first potential problem area deals with specific determiners. There are positive and negative specific determiners. Positive specific determiners include *all*, *every*, *everybody*, *everyone*, *always*, *all the time*, *invariably*, *will certainly*, *will definitely*, *will absolutely*, and *the best.* Negative specific determiners include *none*, *not one*, *nobody*, *no one*, *never*, *at no time*, *will certainly not*, *will definitely not*, *will absolutely not*, *the worst*, and *impossible.* When specific determiners like these are included in an option, that option is *usually incorrect.* These words make statements absolute, and there are few absolutes in the world.

However, some specific determiners are associated with correct statements. Look for more general terms such as *often*, *perhaps*, *seldom*, *generally*, *may*, and *usually.* Life more often reflects statements that use these kinds of words, rather than the absolute terms presented in the previous paragraph. When you are reading the question, circle the specific determiner so you keep careful track of them. Don't ignore them when answering the question.

The second problem area deals with negative terms. It is more difficult to interpret statements that contain negatives than it is to interpret statements without negatives. Here's an example of a double-negative statement: "Donald works well with patients. Therefore it is not untrue to say that he may be a good pharmacy technician." Cross out the *not* and the *un-* and reread the statement. It means the same thing but is easier to understand. Negatives include words such as *no*, *not*, *none*, and *never*, and prefixes such as *il-*, *un-*, and *im-*. Negative prefixes are particularly difficult because they are easily overlooked when reading a statement. Underline negatives in the question so you do not overlook them when answering the question.

Another common trouble area in objective tests is "all or none of the above" questions. One way to confirm the choice of "all of the above" is to find two correct answers among the options. For example, if you are confident that two of the four options are correct, then choosing "all of the above" is a pretty safe bet. Similarly, if you find one that is definitely incorrect, the "all of the above" must be ruled out.

The last type of question that is usually problematic for test takers is the best choice option. The options presented may not contain the correct answer, but possibilities from which you choose the best option. Another way of thinking of it is to think of the correct option as the least problematic. Select your answer by a process of elimination.

Mental Blocks

You know you know the material. You've been answering questions—and all of a sudden, you can't seem to think. You have a mental block. One useful technique is to think of the multiple-choice question as a series of true and false statements. In other words, make statements or complete sentences out of each of the options and then ask yourself if the statement is true or false. This change in perspective may help you to answer a difficult question or just refresh your thinking processes. However, keep your time limitations in mind and don't spend too much time on any one question. Skip difficult questions and come back to them, or take a quick 1-minute mental break to refresh yourself.

Final Review

Always plan on saving time to review your test before handing it in to the proctor. Check your math if any of the questions required calculations. Contrary to popular belief, research has shown that test takers generally increase their scores when they review their answers and make changes. Make changes thoughtfully, though. When changing an answer, make sure you have taken into consideration the reasons why you answered the questions the way you did in the first place.

Finally, don't let other test takers distract you; concentrate on what you are doing. Do not be concerned if other people are finishing the exam before you. They may be finishing early because they simply are not as prepared as you are and therefore cannot answer all the questions. There is little relationship between the amount of time spent on a test and the test scores.

Coping with Test Anxieties

At the beginning of this chapter, we discussed how many people face taking an exam with dread and anxiety. It has been estimated that half of the nation's students suffer test anxiety, and one-quarter of them are significantly hampered by it.[1] You may feel faint at heart, apprehensive, nervous, nauseated, dizzy, or even have heart palpitations. Some people describe it as "my mind goes blank." Some amount of test anxiety is normal, so you just need to learn how to make it work for you. The first step is to recognize that some anxiety is natural; it serves as a primary motivator in your performance.

There are three components of test anxiety. The first one is fear of failure. Nobody likes to fail, but remember to keep it in perspective. Tests just measure and assess one aspect of your life. Passing or failing a test reflects your performance in one area at one particular time. The second component of test anxiety is the pressure of time. You have a limited amount of time to accomplish a task and to accomplish it as accurately as possible. We all feel the pressure of time in many situations aside from testing. The third component is the logistics of taking the exam. You must read the instructions, follow them, understand the questions, and select the correct answer. Generally, the higher the stakes, the more anxiety you may feel, particularly if the competition is intense.

If your anxiety is moderate, several relaxation techniques are helpful in calming your nerves. Physical relaxation is one technique. First, sit comfortably with both feet on the floor and your hands resting on your thighs. Release all your body tension, close your eyes, and count backward from 10 to 1. Count only on each exhalation and breathe very deeply from the abdomen.[1]

Another physical technique is to clench your hands tightly for 5 to 10 seconds and then slowly relax your hands. Repeat this process throughout the muscles in your entire body. Complete your relaxation exercise by taking a deep breath and tensing your entire body, then relaxing it.

Now that your body is relaxed, try to relax your mind as well. One popular technique is imagining yourself in a peaceful setting. Picture a pleasing situation, such as lying on a favorite beach, sitting in your backyard with the sun shining, or taking a walk in a park or along the lake. When you are feeling particularly stressed, imagine peaceful images.

At all costs, avoid fear-generating thoughts. Do not focus on the negative consequences; instead, focus on the positive outcomes of your examination.

These are just a few simple techniques that may help you relax so that you can do your best. For some, however, test anxiety is so severe that it prevents them from performing at their best. If you experience severe anxiety, you may benefit from seeking personal counseling.

Conclusion

Now that the exam is over, you deserve a reward. Be kind to yourself. However, do spend a few minutes to review what worked for you and what didn't. Think about your preparation. Did you allow yourself enough time? Did you understand what was important to study and learn and what were minor details? How about the test itself? Did you overview the test, run through it several times, and save time for review and checking your answers? One of the most important lessons in life is to learn from your experiences, so evaluate your performance and learn how you can make it better. You may register and take this examination again if you need to. Most likely, there will be other exams in your life as well.

This chapter presented an overview of objective tests, basic study skills, and test-taking strategies. It also presented some simple techniques for relaxation to refresh you. But remember, no matter how effective the strategies, there is no substitute for adequate and thorough preparation. Begin your preparation early, be organized, use small increments of time, break your studying down into small tasks, and relax.

Suggested Reading

Heiman M, Slomianko J. *Success in College and Beyond.* Allston, MA: Learning to Learn Inc.; 1993.

Pauk W. *How to Study in College.* 9th ed. Boston: Houghton Mifflin; 2007.

Shepherd JF. *College Study Skills.* 6th ed. Boston: Houghton Mifflin; 1998.

Reference

1. Hill KT. Interfering effects of test anxiety on test performance: a growing educational problem and solutions to it. *Ill Sch Res Dev.* 1983;20:8–19.

Chapter 7

Practice Exam

Choose the *best* answer for each of the following questions.

1. Information that is generally *not* found in a patient's profile in an outpatient pharmacy includes which of the following?
   a. preferences regarding child-resistant packaging
   b. date of birth
   c. preferred hospital
   d. prescription and refill history
   e. allergies
2. Which of the following *is not* a part of a syringe?
   a. plunger
   b. Luer-lok tip
   c. bevel
   d. barrel
   e. calibration marks
3. Which abbreviation is *not* used to specify a unit of measure?
   a. hx
   b. oz
   c. kg
   d. ml
   e. tsp
4. What is the *inventory par level*?
   a. the amount of drug that should be purchased at one time
   b. the inventory level at which an order should be placed to prevent running too low
   c. the maximum amount of a particular drug that should be on the shelf at any time
   d. the number generally posted on the shelf label where the drug is stored
   e. b and d
5. Express the following in reduced form: 3/4 + 7/8
   a. 13/8
   b. 2
   c. 1 3/8
   d. 1.5
   e. 1 5/8
6. A child is to be treated with 50 milligrams (mg) of a particular drug per kilograms (kg) of body weight. If the child weighs 38 pounds, what is the dose of the drug that should be administered (round to the nearest 5 mg)?
   a. 430 mg
   b. 865 mg
   c. 1,200 mg
   d. 1,655 mg
   e. 1,900 mg
7. Using the information from the previous question, how much would be needed to provide the correct dose if the drug concentration is 100 mg per milliliter (ml)?
   a. 4.3 ml
   b. 8.65 ml
   c. 12 ml
   d. 16.55 ml
   e. 19 ml
8. Which of the following is *not* a low molecular weight heparin (LMWH)?
   a. heparin

b. enoxaparin
c. dalteparin
d. tinzaparin
e. All of the above are LMWHs.

9. A medication order should contain all of the following elements *except* which one?
a. the dosage form of the product to be dispensed
b. the patient's room number
c. the name of the drug
d. the dose of the drug
e. All of the above should be included.

10. What is *quality control*?
a. a final check to ensure safety and quality of the preparation
b. something done only by the pharmacist
c. something accomplished by comparing the finished product with pictures of what it should look like
d. all of the above
e. none of the above

11. Which of the following should be used to clean the interior of the laminar airflow workbench?
a. 70% isopropyl alcohol
b. 98% ethyl alcohol
c. water and a lint-free cloth
d. 50% acetone
e. a and c

12. Which of the following is (are) used to describe a needle?
a. bevel
b. shaft length
c. gauge
d. all of the above
e. none of the above

13. Which statement(s) is (are) true of the Internet?
a. It contains only reputable sources.
b. It can be used to access on-line versions of many of the popular print references.
c. It should be recommended to computer-using patients instead of offering patient counseling.
d. It is a good place to look for general information about diseases, such as contacting support groups.
e. b and d

14. Which abbreviation stands for "before meals"?
a. hs
b. pc
c. tid
d. qd
e. ac

15. Which of the following is *false* concerning the drug receiving process in a pharmacy?
a. It is not necessary to verify the number of boxes delivered.
b. Each item should be carefully checked to make sure it is the correct drug and correct strength.
c. Expiration dating should be checked so that short-dated products can be returned.
d. Controlled substances require additional record-keeping steps.
e. The person who checked-in the order should sign the invoice or packing slip.

16. Which of the following is *false* regarding the Poison Prevention Packaging Act?
a. A patient may opt out of the requirements of the act upon request.
b. The act requires all prescriptions to be dispensed in child-resistant packaging, with a few exceptions.
c. One exception to the act is nitroglycerin tablets.
d. A physician specializing in geriatrics may instruct a pharmacy never to use child-resistant packages for any of his prescriptions because all his patients are elderly.
e. The act does not apply to hospital dispensing for inpatients.

17. What is one kg equal to?
a. 1,000 mg
b. 2.2 pounds
c. 10,000 mcg
d. all of the above
e. none of the above

18. A patient is supposed to take 375 mg of an antibiotic three times daily for 10 days. The pharmacy dispenses 250 mg per 5 ml suspension. How much must the patient take per dose?
a. 3.75 ml
b. 5 ml
c. 7.5 ml
d. 8.75 ml
e. 10 ml

19. Using the information from the previous question, how much should the pharmacy dispense for the full 10-day supply?
   a. 100 ml
   b. 150 ml
   c. 200 ml
   d. 225 ml
   e. 300 ml
20. Which of the following is an anticonvulsant?
   a. phenytoin
   b. dexamethasone
   c. amiodarone
   d. hydrochlorothiazide
   e. albuterol
21. Which of the following is *not* used for HIV?
   a. Didanosine
   b. Zidovudine
   c. Nelfinavir
   d. Indinavir
   e. Irbesartan
22. A prescription for a controlled substance includes the DEA number BB1197967. Which of the following is *false* about the DEA number?
   a. The formula for verifying that the DEA number is correct includes adding the first, third, and fifth digits in the number.
   b. The individual to whom this number belongs has a last name that starts with a *B*.
   c. The formula for verifying that the DEA number is correct includes adding the second, fourth, and sixth digits in the number and multiplying by 2.
   d. This number must belong to a pharmacy because it begins with a *B*.
   e. This DEA number is valid.
23. Risks of intravenous (IV) therapy include which of the following?
   a. infection
   b. bleeding
   c. extravasation
   d. air embolus
   e. all of the above
24. Which is the best reference to use to look up whether an IV drug is compatible with a fluid?
   a. *Drug Facts and Comparisons*
   b. *Red Book*
   c. *The Physicians' Desk Reference*
   d. *American Drug Index*
   e. Trissel's *Handbook on Injectable Drugs*
25. Which abbreviation stands for "at bedtime"?
   a. dx
   b. ac
   c. qid
   d. hs
   e. po
26. Which question can a technician answer without involving a pharmacist?
   a. "What is the dose of morphine for a 2-year-old?"
   b. "Is phenytoin compatible with D_5W?"
   c. "I have been feeling dizzy since I started my new medication. Is it possible the drug is causing this feeling?"
   d. "Can I get a TB test if I am pregnant?"
   e. "Is Nuprin® the same thing as ibuprofen?"
27. *Maximizing inventory turns* is which of the following?
   a. a means of minimizing inventory carrying costs
   b. rotating inventory regularly to prevent outdating
   c. the same thing as EOQ
   d. also known as the Minimum Cost Quantity Approach
   e. none of the above
28. Which Controlled Substance Schedule denotes a drug with high abuse potential and no recognized medical use?
   a. Schedule I
   b. Schedule II
   c. Schedule III
   d. Schedule IV
   e. Schedule V
29. Which of the following is true regarding a power of attorney (POA) to sign a DEA Form 222?
   a. The POA can only be assigned to a pharmacist.
   b. The POA can only be assigned to one other person besides the individual whose name is on the license.
   c. The POA must be the pharmacist-in-charge.
   d. The person who signed the original license application can revoke the POA at any time.
   e. It is illegal to assign the POA to anyone to sign the DEA Form 222.

30. Which of the following requires technicians to maintain confidentiality of medical information?
    a. Food, Drug, and Cosmetic Act
    b. Omnibus Reconciliation Act of 1990
    c. Health Insurance Portability and Accountability Act of 1996
    d. Federal Controlled Substance Act
    e. Poison Prevention Packaging Act

31. What is 25% equal to?
    a. 25 out of 100
    b. 0.25
    c. 1/4
    d. all of the above
    e. none of the above

32. Which of the following is the brand name for loratidine?
    a. ChlorTrimeton®
    b. Claritin®
    c. Zyrtec®
    d. Allegra®
    e. Benadryl®

33. Which category of drugs has the characteristic ending "–olol"?
    a. loop diuretics
    b. ACE inhibitors
    c. angiotensin II receptor blockers
    d. beta-blockers
    e. none of the above

34. Which of the following is an *atypical* antipsychotic?
    a. Haloperidol
    b. Fluphenazine
    c. Chlorpromazine
    d. Risperidone
    e. Loxapine

35. Considerations in determining the stability of compounded preparations include all of the following *except* which one?
    a. light sensitivity
    b. container in which the product is stored
    c. time of day when the product is prepared
    d. physical characteristics of the finished product
    e. chemical characteristics of the finished product

36. Which is the best reference to use to look up information that would appear in a manufacturer's package insert?
    a. *Drug Facts and Comparisons*
    b. *Red Book*
    c. *The Physicians' Desk Reference*
    d. *American Drug Index*
    e. Trissel's *Handbook on Injectable Drugs*

37. Which of the following is *false* regarding prescription transfer?
    a. Transfer of a prescription from one pharmacy to another can be done over the phone.
    b. A technician may be involved in one side of a transfer phone call as long as a pharmacist is involved on the other end of the line.
    c. If no refills remain on a prescription, it may not be transferred and filled without contacting the physician.
    d. Transfers are easier if the patient brings the prescription bottle to the pharmacy that will be receiving the prescription.
    e. Once a prescription has been transferred, the original pharmacy must no longer refill the prescription.

38. Which abbreviation stands for "ointment"?
    a. oz
    b. OTC
    c. pr
    d. ung
    e. kg

39. Which question should be referred to a pharmacist?
    a. "Who manufactures Lovenox®?"
    b. "How much codeine is in one Tylenol #3® tablet?"
    c. "What is the difference in price between brand name Darvocet N-100® and the generic version?"
    d. "If I am allergic to penicillin, is it safe for me to take erythromycin?"
    e. "How long is the shortage of Zemuron® likely to last?"

40. Calculate the inventory turnover rate if the pharmacy's purchases for the past year were $14,845,222 and the inventory as of December 31 was $655,879 (round to the nearest whole number).
    a. 16 times
    b. 23 times
    c. 12 times
    d. 19 times
    e. 35 times

41. In which Controlled Substance Schedule does morphine belong?
   a. Schedule I
   b. Schedule II
   c. Schedule III
   d. Schedule IV
   e. Schedule V

42. All the following must be included in patient counseling according to the Omnibus Reconciliation Act of 1990 (OBRA 90) *except* which one?
   a. the name of the medication
   b. whether a generic version is available
   c. proper storage
   d. the route of administration
   e. common side effects

43. If you are to prepare an IV fluid with 2 grams of magnesium sulfate using a solution with 500 mg of magnesium sulfate per ml, how many ml do you need?
   a. 1.25 ml
   b. 2 ml
   c. 3.5 ml
   d. 4 ml
   e. 5 ml

44. Which of the following is *not* a known side effect of the tricyclic antidepressants?
   a. dry mouth
   b. constipation
   c. frequent urination
   d. blurred vision
   e. sedation

45. Which vitamin is fat-soluble?
   a. B-vitamins
   b. vitamin C
   c. vitamin D
   d. vitamin E
   e. c and d

46. Common error messages received from third-party payers include all of the following *except* which one?
   a. refill too late
   b. refill too soon
   c. invalid patient ID
   d. drug-drug interaction
   e. nonformulary or medication not covered

47. Which of the following is true regarding the use of a laminar airflow workbench?
   a. Objects brought into the hood should be lined up from the back of the hood to the front to create the least turbulence.
   b. No work should be done within six inches from the front of the hood.
   c. Syringes should always be aimed toward the HEPA filter to avoid spraying out into the room.
   d. Objects that are not in use in the hood should be placed against either wall to keep them out of the way.
   e. The zone of turbulence around an object is roughly five times the size of the object.

48. Which is the best reference to use to look up a price?
   a. *Drug Facts and Comparisons*
   b. *Red Book*
   c. *The Physicians' Desk Reference*
   d. *American Drug Index*
   e. Trissel's *Handbook on Injectable Drugs*

49. How many 10 ml doses can be packaged from a pint of medication (round down to the nearest 10 ml increment)?
   a. 24
   b. 35
   c. 47
   d. 75
   e. 100

50. Which abbreviation stands for "four times daily"?
   a. ac
   b. qid
   c. po
   d. prn
   e. stat

51. Which of the following corresponds to "refrigerated" by USP standards?
   a. 2° to 8°C
   b. 68° to 77°F
   c. 36° to 46°F
   d. 8° to 15°C
   e. a and c

52. Which of the following are examples of automated dispensing machines?
   a. Pyxis®
   b. Omnicell®

c. SureMed®
d. Meditrol®
e. all of the above

53. Which of the following is true concerning drug samples?
    a. Pharmacies may order drug samples as long as they sign an agreement not to charge patients for them.
    b. Drug samples do not require any special handling or record-keeping.
    c. It is necessary to maintain logs with receiving and dispensing information for all samples.
    d. It is acceptable to charge a small handling fee for samples to pay for the extra record-keeping that is required.
    e. none of the above

54. Which Controlled Substance Schedule denotes a drug with the least abuse potential?
    a. Schedule I
    b. Schedule II
    c. Schedule III
    d. Schedule IV
    e. Schedule V

55. Routine maintenance of the sterile compounding area should include which of the following?
    a. The laminar airflow workbench prefilter should be changed at least weekly.
    b. Cardboard should not be allowed in the area.
    c. The HEPA filter should be changed every six months.
    d. The laminar airflow workbench should be cleaned at least every hour during use.
    e. Hood cleaning should be done from "dirty" to "clean" to avoid contamination.

56. What is one teaspoon equal to?
    a. 1/2 tablespoon
    b. 10 ml
    c. 5 ml
    d. 1/3 tablespoon
    e. c and d

57. Which of the following antihyperlipidemics is classified as a fibrate?
    a. fluvastatin
    b. nicotinic acid
    c. gemfibrozil
    d. cholestyramine
    e. none of the above

58. Which proton pump inhibitor is available as an injectable product?
    a. Omeprazole
    b. Pantoprazole
    c. Lansoprazole
    d. Rabeprazole
    e. Both b and c

59. What volume would deliver 50 mg if the solution contains 12.5 mg/ml?
    a. 2 ml
    b. 3 ml
    c. 4 ml
    d. 5 ml
    e. none of the above

60. Key areas of good compounding practices include which of the following?
    a. maintaining the compounding environment
    b. quality control
    c. ingredient selection
    d. stability of compounded preparations
    e. all of the above

61. What are Material Safety Data Sheets?
    a. sheets used by technicians to get information about hazardous chemicals
    b. sheets that contain information about how to handle a drug safely
    c. sheets that list physical and chemical properties of the drugs
    d. sheets that provide information on how to treat an exposure
    e. all of the above

62. Which abbreviation stands for "drop"?
    a. dr
    b. OD
    c. qod
    d. gtt
    e. g

63. Which question should be referred to a pharmacist?
    a. "What is the brand name of Zoloft®?"
    b. "Should amoxicillin suspension be kept in the refrigerator?"
    c. "What is the usual dose of ciprofloxacin?"
    d. "How many milliliters are in a teaspoonful?"
    e. "Is Claritin® available over the counter?"

64. Which of the following require special storage considerations?
   a. look-alike/sound-alike drugs
   b. controlled substances
   c. investigational drugs
   d. chemotherapy drugs
   e. all of the above

65. What is the *economic order quantity*?
   a. a model for calculating inventory order quantities
   b. also known as the *minimum cost quantity approach*
   c. the least amount of a drug that it is economical for the manufacturer to package for sale
   d. both a and b
   e. both a and c

66. In which Controlled Substance Schedule do the benzodiazepine drugs belong?
   a. Schedule I
   b. Schedule II
   c. Schedule III
   d. Schedule IV
   e. Schedule V

67. The Omnibus Reconciliation Act of 1990 (OBRA 90) requires which of the following?
   a. that pharmacies that receive federal reimbursement for prescriptions (Medicare/Medicaid) offer counseling to patients getting prescriptions filled
   b. that the pharmacist personally make the offer to counsel patients
   c. that all patients be counseled about their prescriptions
   d. that someone in the pharmacy counsel patients, including a technician, if that person happens to be available and the pharmacist is not
   e. none of the above

68. Convert the fraction to a decimal number: 3/4
   a. 0.25
   b. 0.5
   c. 0.75
   d. 0.67
   e. 0.34

69. Which of the following is a potassium-sparing diuretic?
   a. Chlorthalidone
   b. Spironolactone
   c. Furosemide
   d. Triamterene
   e. both b and d

70. All of the following are reasons to give medications by the IV route, *except* which one?
   a. Drug characteristics make it impossible for the medication to be given by any other route.
   b. Patient is unable to take the medication by any other route.
   c. IV administration is desired for a quicker onset of action.
   d. Some medications cause pain at the injection site.
   e. all of the above

71. If you have to make 100 ml of a 10% w/v solution from water and a 90% w/v solution, how much of the 90% solution do you need to use?
   a. 9 ml
   b. 10 ml
   c. 11 ml
   d. 12 ml
   e. none of the above

72. Which of the following are appropriate for clean room attire?
   a. low-lint clothing
   b. no jewelry on the hands or wrists
   c. hair covers
   d. shoe covers
   e. all of the above

73. Which of the following drugs *does not* belong in Schedule II?
   a. cocaine
   b. morphine
   c. propoxyphine
   d. fentanyl
   e. a and c

74. If you have to mix a KCl infusion with 35 mEq of KCl using a vial of KCl with 40 mEq in 20 ml, how much volume do you need to add?
   a. 3.5 ml
   b. 10 ml
   c. 12.5 ml
   d. 17.5 ml
   e. 20 ml

75. Which insulin is classified as rapid acting?
   a. Lispro®
   b. Lantus®
   c. Levemir®
   d. NPH®

76. Which of the following does not belong?
    a. Zebeta
    b. Lopressor
    c. Tenormin
    d. Procardia
    e. Inderal
77. If a drug is ordered "one pc & hs" and 40 capsules are dispensed, what is the estimated days supply?
    a. 10
    b. 12
    c. 15
    d. 40
78. How many grams of hydrocortisone would be required to make one pound of a 5% ointment?
    a. 2.27 g
    b. 3 g
    c. 5 g
    d. 22.7 g
    e. 90.8 g
79. Convert 180 lb to kg.
    a. 81.8 kg
    b. 100 kg
    c. 120 kg
    d. 396 kg
80. Adderall® is a
    a. schedule II drug
    b. schedule III drug
    c. schedule IV drug
    d. schedule V drug
    e. not a scheduled drug
81. Which DEA number listed below is valid for Dr. Maxine Smith?
    a. AM 4561937
    b. AS 4561937
    c. BM 4561937
    d. BS 4561933
    e. AB 4561933
82. If a patient is taking an antitussive they are treating
    a. an allergy
    b. a productive cough
    c. a dry non-productive cough
    d. congestion
    e. post nasal drip
83. Which set of NDC numbers represents the manufacturer of the product?
    a. the first set
    b. the second set
    c. the third set
    d. none of them represent the manufacturer
84. Which strength would represent the most dilute drug product?
    a. 25%
    b. 2.5%
    c. 0.25%
    d. 0.025%
85. Which drug category is *not* covered by Medicare Part D?
    a. antidepressants
    b. benzodiazepines
    c. HIV drugs
    d. antipsychotics
    e. cancer agents
86. Medicare Part A
    a. covers hospital, skilled nursing facilities, hospice care, and some home health
    b. is an optional insurance for outpatient and hospital services, clinical lab services, and durable medical equipment
    c. is the Medicare Advantage plan which includes HMOs and PPOs
    d. is the federal prescription drug program
    e. covers low-income Americans and the disabled
87. If a medication contains 160 mg of drug per teaspoon, how many grams of medication would be in a 4 oz. bottle?
    a. 3840 g
    b. 38.4 g
    c. 3.84 g
    d. 1280 g
    e. 1.28 g
88. Why would a patient be taking pantoprazole?
    a. they have GERD
    b. they suffer from depression
    c. they have high cholesterol
    d. they have high blood pressure
    e. they suffer from OCD
89. How many refills may be ordered for Vicodin®?
    a. no refills may be ordered
    b. limited to 5 refills in a 6 month time period
    c. limited to 6 refills in a 5 month time period

d. may be refilled as often as the doctor orders, up to a year

90. What agency licenses pharmacies, investigates complaints, and provides disciplinary action against pharmacist and pharmacy technicians?
    a. DEA
    b. NABP
    c. FDA
    d. state boards of pharmacy
    e. ASHP

91. The Restricted Drug Distribution System (RDDS)
    a. ensures that investigational drugs are dispensed in accordance to the FDA standards.
    b. ensures that controlled drugs are stored within DEA standards.
    c. ensures that drugs identified as "high risk" are safely procured, prescribed, dispensed and administered.
    d. ensures that all medication dispensed complies with the Poison Prevention Act.

92. Which category of drugs has the characteristic "*artan*" ending?
    a. ACE inhibitors
    b. ARBs
    c. Beta Blockers
    d. benzodiazepines
    e. none of the above

93. Convert 1:20000 to a %.
    a. 0.00005%
    b. 0.005%
    c. 0.05%
    d. 0.5%
    e. 5%

94. The official order form for each distribution, purchase or transfer of a schedule II substance is
    a. DEA Form 227.
    b. DEA Form 222.
    c. CSA Form 222.
    d. PDR Form 227.

95. Calculate the flow rate for 1 liter of IV fluid to run in over 12 hours using a set calibrated to deliver 10 gtt/mL.
    a. 7 gtts/min
    b. 13 gtts/min
    c. 14 gtts/min
    d. 833 gtts/min

96. The pharmacy has 10 grams of codeine in stock. The following products have been made using this supply:
    1. 30 capsules each containing 30 mg of codeine
    2. 6 oz. of cough suppressant containing 15 mg/tsp
    3. 16 oz. of medication containing 45mg/tsp

    How many grams of codeine are remaining?
    a. 4.24 g
    b. 0.424 g
    c. 7.48 g
    d. 0.748 g

97. 75 mg of a drug is ordered in 250 mL of fluid. This is to infuse at 2 mcg/kg/min for a patient weighing 150 lb. Calculate the flow rate in mL/hr.
    a. 2 mL/hr
    b. 20 mL/hr
    c. 27 mL/hr
    d. 200 mL/hr

98. The generic name of Lexapro® is
    a. estramustine
    b. citalopram
    c. eszopiclone
    d. escitalopram

99. Why would a patient be taking alendronate?
    a. they have high blood pressure
    b. they are suffering from glaucoma
    c. they have osteoporosis
    d. they suffer from allergies

100. The generic name of Lipitor® is
    a. simvastatin
    b. pravastatin
    c. lovastatin
    d. atorvastatin
    e. rouvastatin

101. A patient taking furosemide may need to
    a. increase their chloride intake.
    b. eat foods rich in calcium.
    c. increase their potassium intake by eating foods high in potassium or supplements.
    d. all the above.

102. Which of the following is used to treat erectile dysfunction?
    a. silfenafil
    b. donepezil
    c. enalapril
    d. gemfibrozil

103. What is the brand name for gabapentin?
   a. Metformin®
   b. Cymbalta®
   c. Namenda®
   d. Neurontin®

104. Which of the following is stored with the C-II medications?
   a. methylphenidate
   b. oxytocin
   c. Lortab®
   d. Lunesta®

105. The pharmacy has 250 mL of a 35% solution. 100 mL of diluent was added. How many grams of medication are in the diluted product?
   a. 25 g
   b. 40 g
   c. 87.5 g
   d. 218.75 g

106. If you add 15 g of coal tar to one pound of a 5% coal tar ointment, what is the % strength of the final product?
   a. 3.8%
   b. 5%
   c. 8%
   d. 126%

107. In what proportion should zinc oxide be mixed with a 25% product to make a 40% zinc oxide product?
   a. 1:10
   b. 1:6
   c. 1:5
   d. 1:4

108. If a medication is ordered at 5 mg/kg per day and the patient weighs 65 lb., how many grams will the patient receive if the mediation is taken 10 days?
   a. 1.477 g
   b. 14.77g
   c. 6.05 g
   d. 605 g
   e. 6,050 g

109. The brand name for lorazepam is
   a. Ativan®
   b. Claritin®
   c. Xanax®
   d. Klonopin®

110. Which drug must be dispensed in its original easy-open container?
   a. Imitrex SL
   b. nitroglycerin SL
   c. diazepam
   d. propranolol

111. A patient who is prescribed Lantus® has
   a. glaucoma
   b. Alzheimer disease
   c. CHF
   d. diabetes
   e. Parkinson disease

112. The generic name of Abilify® is
   a. primidone
   b. fluconazole
   c. aripiprazole
   d. econazole

113. Ciprofloxacin is
   a. a penicillin antibiotic
   b. a cephalosporin antibiotic
   c. a fluoroquinolone antibiotic
   d. a macrlolide antibiotic

114. A patient taking citalopram
   a. is suffering from depression
   b. is suffering from a fungal infection
   c. is suffering from an allergy
   d. is suffering from GERD

115. Which pair listed below would be an example of duplication of therapy?
   a. Protonix®/Prevacid®
   b. nitroglycerin/digoxin
   c. Actos®/Videx®
   d. Levaquin®/ciprofloxacin

116. How many 125 mg doses are available in 75 mL of a suspension marked 250 mg/5 mL?
   a. 10
   b. 15
   c. 20
   d. 30

117. At what standard time should a patient receive their medication if the order says to give it at 1800 hours military time?
   a. 4 PM
   b. 5 PM
   c. 6 PM
   d. 8 PM

118. Which option is the best choice for the prescription label directions if the prescription reads "*Amoxicillin 400/5 Sig: 600mg po BID X 10 days*"?
   a. take 600 mg twice a day for 10 days
   b. take 7.5 mL twice a day for 10 days
   c. take 1½ teaspoonful by mouth twice a day for 10 days
   d. take 1½ teaspoonful by mouth daily for 10 days

119. Using the information in question 118, how many milliliters must be dispensed?
   a. 100 mL
   b. 150 mL
   c. 200 mL
   d. 250 mL

120. How many minutes should the blower on a laminar airflow workbench be allowed to run prior to use?
   a. 10–20 min
   b. 15–30 min
   c. 30–60 min
   d. no less than 60 min

121. Which drug listed below is *not* an SSRI?
   a. Celexa®
   b. Paxil®
   c. Zoloft®
   d. Lexapro®
   e. Cymbalta®

122. Why would a patient be taking Aricept®?
   a. they have osteoporosis
   b. they have Alzheimer disease
   c. they have Parkinson disease
   d. they have high blood pressure
   e. they have CHF

123. You are to make two ounces of a solution containing 15 mg/5mL and your stock solution that you have on hand is 5 mg/mL. How much drug and how much diluent do you need?
   a. 36 mL of drug; 24 mL of diluent
   b. 24 mL of drug; 36 mL of diluent
   c. 90 mL of drug; 40 mL of diluent
   d. 40 mL of drug; 90 mL of diluent

124. How many grams of drug are in 2 liters of a 15% solution?
   a. 300 g
   b. 150 g
   c. 3000 g
   d. 30,000 g

125. Which drug is available OTC?
   a. Singulair®
   b. Spiriva®
   c. Zyrtec®
   d. Allegra®
   e. hydroxyzine

Answer Key

1. c
2. c
3. a
4. c
5. e
6. b
7. b
8. a
9. e
10. a
11. e
12. d
13. e
14. e
15. a
16. d
17. b
18. c
19. d
20. a
21. e
22. d
23. e
24. e
25. d
26. e
27. a
28. a
29. d
30. c
31. d
32. b
33. d
34. d
35. c
36. c
37. b
38. d
39. d
40. b
41. b
42. b
43. d
44. c
45. e
46. a
47. b
48. b
49. c
50. b
51. e
52. e
53. c
54. e
55. b
56. c
57. c
58. e
59. c
60. e
61. e
62. d
63. c
64. e
65. d
66. d
67. a
68. c

Answer Key

69. e
70. d
71. c
72. e
73. c
74. d
75. a
76. d
77. a
78. d
79. a
80. a
81. b
82. c
83. a
84. d
85. b
86. a
87. c
88. a
89. b
90. d
91. c
92. b
93. b
94. b
95. c
96. a
97. c
98. d
99. c
100. d
101. c
102. a
103. d
104. a
105. c
106. c
107. d
108. a
109. a
110. b
111. d
112. c
113. c
114. a
115. d
116. d
117. c
118. c
119. b
120. b
121. e
122. b
123. a
124. a
125. c

Appendix A

Medical Terminology and Abbreviations

Familiarity with and understanding medical terms and abbreviations is critical to the success of a pharmacy technician because it can help the technician be more helpful and productive.

Learning medical terminology may seem like learning a whole new language. Most medical terms, however, are built from component parts, called word roots, prefixes, and suffixes. The root is the base component of the word, which is modified by the addition of a prefix or suffix. Prefixes are modifying components placed in front of the word root. Examples include pre-, post-, and sub-. Suffixes appear at the end of the word root and are connected to the root by a combining vowel, for example, -ism, -itis, -ous. Combining vowels (most often “o”) are often used to link roots to suffixes and to join roots when a term includes more than one root. These combining vowels are often shown along with the root as a combining form, as in “bronch/o.”

The process of defining a medical term starts with identifying and defining the components and then combining those definitions into a coherent whole. For example, consider the word *bronchoscopy.* First, divide the word into its components: “bronch/o” and “-scopy.” Then, define each of the parts: *bronch/o* means bronchus, and *-scopy* means the process of viewing. Therefore, bronchoscopy means the process of viewing the bronchus.

What is the definition of *electrocardiogram?* First, break the word into its parts: “electro-,” “cardi/o,” and “-gram.” Second, define each part: *electro-* means electricity, *cardi/o* means heart, and *-gram* means record. Finally, put the definitions together to get the complete definition of the word: recording the electrical activity of the heart.

Tables A-1, A-2, and **A-3** include the meanings of many of the most common word roots, prefixes, and suffixes. Familiarity with these component parts will help you understand medical terminology.

After you have reviewed the meanings of the component parts, read through the common medical terms by body system. Each term is accompanied by its pronunciation and definition and by an analysis of term structure.

Table A-1. Prefixes

Prefix	Meaning
a-; an-; ana-	no; not; without
ab-	away from
ante-	before; forward
anti-	against
auto-	self
bi-	two; double; both
brady-	slow
carcin-	cancerous
contra-	against; opposite
dys-	difficult; painful
ect-	outside; out
en-	within; in
endo-	within
epi-	above; upon
ex-	out
gynec/o-	woman
hemi-	half
hyper-	above; excessive
hypo-	below; deficient
infra-	below; inferior
inter-	between
intra-	within
iso-	same; equal
macro-	large
mal-	bad; poor; abnormal
meta-	change; after; beyond
micro-	small
multi-	many
neo-	new
non-	not
oligo-	few; less
pan-	all
para-	near; beside
per-	through
peri-	around; surrounding
poly-	many; excessive
post-	after
pre-	before; in front of
primi-	first
retro-	behind; backward; upward

Prefix	Meaning
semi-	half
sub-	below; under
super-	above; over; excess
supra-	above; on top of
sym-	with
syn-	together; with
tachy-	fast
tri-	three
uni-	one
xero-	dry

Table A-2. Suffixes

Suffix	Meaning
-ac; -al; -ar; -ary	pertaining to
-algia	pain
-blast	germ or bud
-cele	hernia; herniation
-centesis	surgical puncture
-crine	to secrete
-crit	to separate
-cyte	cell
-cytosis	condition of cells
-desis	binding together
-ectomy	surgical removal; excision
-emesis	vomit
-emia	blood
-genesis; -genic; -gen	origin; producing; forming
-globin; -globulin	protein
-gram	record
-graph	instrument for recording
-graphy	process of recording
-ia; -iac; -ic	pertaining to
-iasis	formation or presence of
-ism	condition
-itis	inflammation
-ium	structure or tissue
-lepsy	seizure
-lysis; -lytic	break down
-malacia	softening

Table A-2. Suffixes (continued)

Suffix	Meaning
-megaly	enlargement
-oid	resembling; like
-(o)logist	specialist in the study or treatment of
-(o)logy	study of
-oma	tumor
-osis	abnormal condition
-ostomy	creation of an opening
-otomy	incision into
-ous	pertaining to
-paresis	paralysis
-pathy	disease
-penia	decreased number
-pepsia	digestion
-pexy	suspension or fixation
-phagia	eating; swallowing
-phobia	abnormal fear
-phonia	voice; sound
-phoresis	carrying; transmission
-phoria	feeling; mental state
-plasty	surgical repair
-plegia	paralysis
-pnea	breathing
-poiesis	formation
-r/rhage; -r/rhagia	bursting forth
-rrhea	flow; discharge
-rhexis	rupture
-sclerosis	hardening
-scope	instrument for viewing
-scopy	process of viewing
-somnia	sleep
-spasm	involuntary contraction or twitch
-stasis	control; stop
-stenosis	narrowing
-therapy	treatment
-thorax	chest; pleural cavity
-tocia	labor; birth
-tripsy	crushing
-trophy	growth; development
-tropin	nourish; develop; stimulate

Table A-3. Word Roots

Root	Meaning
abdomin/o	abdomen
aden/o	gland
adip/o	fat
amnio	amnion
andr/o	male; man
angi/o	vessel
aque/o	watery
arteri/o	artery
arteriol/o	arteriole
arthr/o	joint
ather/o	fat; fatty plaque
audi/o	hearing; sound
aur/o	ear
bili	bile; gall
blephar/o	eyelid
bronch/o	bronchus
bronchiol/o	bronchiole
bucc/o	cheek
burs/o	joint
calc/i	calcium
capnia	carbon dioxide
carcin/o	cancer
cardi/o	heart
carp/o	wrist bones
cephal/o	head
cerebr/o	cerebrum
cirrh/o	yellow
chol/e	bile; gall bladder
cholangi/o	bile duct
cholecyst/o	gall bladder
chondr/o	cartilage
coagul/o	clotting
cochle/o	cochlea
col/o	colon
colp/o	vagina (sheath)
conjuctiv/o	conjunctiva
cor/o	heart
corne/o	cornea
coron/o	heart
cost/o	rib

Table A-3. Word Roots (continued)

Root	Meaning
crani/o	cranium; skull
cry/o	cold
cut/o; cuti; cutane/o	skin
cyan/o	blue
cyst/o	bladder; sac
cyt/o	cell
dacry/o	tears
dent	tooth
derm/o; dermat/o	skin
dipl/o	two; double
dips/o	thirst
duoden/o	duodenum
dur/a	dura mater
electr/o	electricity
embry/o	embryo
encephal/o	brain
enter/o	intestines
eosin/o	red cell
epididym/o	epididymis
episi/o	vulva
erythr/o	red
esophag/o	esophagus
esthesi/o	sensation
fasci/o	fascia
femor/o	femur
fet/o; fet/i	fetus
fibul/o	fibula
fund/o	fundus
gastr/o	stomach
gingiv/o	gums
glauc/o	silver; gray
gli/o	nerve cell
glomerul/o	glomerulus
gloss/o	tongue
gluc/o glyc/o	glucose; sugar
gonad/o	sex glands
gravid/a; gravid/o	pregnancy
gyn/o; gyn/e; gynec/o	woman
hemat/o; hem/o	blood
hemangi/o	blood vessel

Table A-3. (continued)

Root	Meaning
hepat/o	liver
hidr/o	sweat
hormone/o	hormone; an urging on
humer/o	humerus
hydr/o	water; fluid
hyster/o	uterus
ile/o; ili/o	ileum
immune/o	protection
jejun/o	jejunum
kal/i	potassium
kerat/o	cornea
ket/o; keton/o	ketone bodies
kinesi/o	movement
lacrim/o	tears
lact/o	milk
lapar/o	abdominal wall
laryng/o	larynx
ligament/o	ligament
lingua	tongue
lip/o	fat
lith/o	stone
lumb/o	lower back
lymph/o	lymph
mamm/o; mast/o	breast
melan/o	black
men/o	menses; menstruation
mening/o; meningi/o	meninges (membrane)
metacarp/o	hand bones
metatars/o	foot bones
morph/o	form; shape
muc/o	mucus
my/o	muscle
myc/o	fungus
myel/o	bone marrow; spinal cord
myring/o	eardrum
narc/o	sleep
nas/o	nose
nat/o; natal	birth; delivery
nephr/o	kidney
neur/o	nerve

Table A-3. Word Roots (continued)

Root	Meaning
noct/o; nyctal/o	night
ocul/o; ophthalm/o; opt/o	eye
onych/o	nail
oophor/o	ovary
or/o	mouth
orch/o; orchi/o; orchid/o	testis; testicle
orth/o	straight
oste/o	bone
ot/o	ear
ovari/o	ovary
oxi	oxygen
pachy/o	thick
pancreat/o	pancreas
par/o; part/o	bear; labor; childbirth
patell/o	kneecap
pector/o	chest
ped	children
pelv/i	pelvis
perine/o	perineum
peritone/o	peritoneum
phag/o	eat or swallow
phalang/o	finger and toe bones
pharyng/o	pharynx
phleb/o	vein
phot/o	light
phren/o	mind or diaphragm
pil/o	hair
pneum/o	lungs; air
pod/o; podi	foot
presby/o	old age
proct/o	rectum
psych/o; psych/i	mind or soul
pub/o	pubis; pubic bone
pulmon/o	lungs
py/o	pus
pyel/o	renal pelvis
quadr/i	four
radi/o	radius

Table A-3. (continued)

Root	Meaning
rect/o	rectum
ren/o	kidney
reticul/o	a net
retin/o	retina
rhabdomy/o	skeletal muscle; striated muscle
rheum	watery discharge
rhin/o	nose
salping/o	eustachian or uterine tube
sarc/o	flesh
schiz/o	split
semin/o	semen
septi	bacteria
sial/o	saliva
sinus/o	sinus
somat/o	body
sperm/o; spermat/o	sperm
spher/o	round
sphygm/o	pulse
spir/o	breathe; breath
splen/o	spleen
spondyl/o	vertebra; vertebral column
steth/o	chest
stoma; stomat/o	mouth
synovi/o	joint
tars/o	ankle bones
ten/o; tend/o;	tendon/o;
tendin/o	tendon
test/o; testicul/o	testis; testicle
thorac/o	chest
thromb/o	clot
thyr/o	thyroid gland
trache/o	trachea
tympan/o	eardrum
urethr/o	urethra
ur/o	urinary tract
vas/o; vascul/o	vessel
ven/o	vein
xanth/o	yellow

Common Medical Terms and Definitions by Body System

General Terms

Term	Phonetic Spelling	Term Structure	Definition
abnormal	ab-'nor-məl	ab = away from normal = conforming to a type, standard, or regular pattern	Deviating from the normal or average
aqueduct	'a-kwə-dəkt	aque/o = watery duct = A tubular structure giving exit to the secretion of a gland or organ: capable of conducting fluid	A conduit or canal
bilateral	bī-'la-t(ə-)rəl	bi = two; double; both lateral = on the side; farther from the median or midsagittal plane	Relating to, or having, two sides
cryolysis	kri'o-lī-'sis	cry/o = cold lysis = break down	Destruction by cold
cyanosis	sī-ə-nō'-səs	cyan/o = blue osis = abnormal condition	A dark bluish or purplish discoloration of the skin and mucous membrane due to deficient oxygenation of the blood
fasciectomy	fas"e-ek'tə-me	fasci/o = fascia ectomy = surgical removal; excision	Excision of strips of fascia
fundusectomy	fun"də-sek'tə-me	fund/o = fundus ectomy = surgical removal; excision	Excision of the fundus of an organ
hidropoiesis	hi"dro-poi-e'sis	hidr/o = sweat poiesis = formation	The formation of sweat
piloid	pī"loid	pil/o = hair oid = resembling; like	Hairlike; resembling hair
preoperative	prē-ä'-p(ə-)rə-tiv	pre = before; in front of operative = relating to or effected by means of an operation	Preceding an operation
pyocyanogenic	pi"-o-si"ə-no-jen'ik	py/o = pus cyan/o = blue genic = origin; producing; forming	Causing blue pus
semilunar	se-mī-lū'-nər	semi = half lunar = moon ar = pertaining to	Pertaining to a half-moon shape
unilateral	yü-ni-la'-tə-rəl	uni = one lateral = on the side	Confined to one side only
venostomy	ve-nos'tə-me	ven/o = vein ostomy = creation of an opening	Dissection of a vein or artery for insertion of a cannula or needle for the administration of intravenous fluids or medication or for measurement of pressure

Nervous System

Term	Phonetic Spelling	Term Structure	Definition
akinesia	a″kĭ-ne′zhə	a = not; without kinesi/o = movement	Loss of normal muscle movement
cerebrospinal	ser″ə-bro-spi′nəl	cerebr/o = cerebrum spin/o = spine al = pertaining to	Pertaining to the brain and the spinal cord
cerebrovascular	ser″ə-bro-vas′ku-lər	cerebr/o = cerebrum vascul/o = vessel spin/o = spine ar = pertaining to	Pertaining to the brain and blood vessels that supply it
electroencephalogram	e-lek″tro-en-sef′ə-lo-gram″	electr/o = electricity encephal/o = brain gram = record	Record of the electrical activity of the brain
epidural	ep″ĭ-doo′rəl	epi = above; upon dur/a = dura mater al = pertaining to	Pertaining to above the dura mater
epilepsy	ep′ĭ-lep″se	epi = upon lepsy = seizure	A disorder of the central nervous system characterized by recurrent seizures
euphoria	u-for′e-ə	eu = good or normal phoria = feeling; mental state	A feeling of well-being
glioblast	gli′-o-blast	gli/o = nerve cell blast = germ or bud	An early neural cell developing
hemiparesis	hem″ĭ-pə-re′sis	hemi = half paresis = paralysis	Paralysis of one side of the body
hydrocephalus	hi″dro-sef′ə-ləs	hydr/o = water; fluid cephal/o = head	Excess cerebrospinal fluid in the brain
hyperesthesia	hi″pər-es-the′zhə	hyper = above or excessive esthesi/o = sensation ia = condition of	Increased sensitivity to stimulation such as touch, pain, and other sensory stimuli
meningitis	men″in-ji′tis	mening/o = meninges itis = inflammation	Inflammation of the meninges of the brain
myelogram	mi′ə-lo-gram	myel/o = bone marrow or spinal cord gram = record	An X-ray of the spinal cord and nerve roots
neuralgia	nōō-ral′jə	neur/o = nerve algia = pain	Nerve pain
neurologist	nōō-rol′ə-jist	neur/o = nerve logist = specialist in the study or treatment of	A physician who specializes in diseases of the neurological system
paraplegia	par″ə-ple′jə	para = near; beside plegia = paralysis	Paralysis of both lower extremities and, generally, the lower trunk
polyneuritis	pol″e-nōō-ri′tis	poly = many or excessive neur/o = nerve itis = inflammation	Inflammation of two or more nerves
polysomnography	pol″e-som-nog′-rə-fe	poly = many; excessive somn/o = sleep graphy = process of recording	The process of recording and evaluating sleep

Nervous System (continued)

Term	Phonetic Spelling	Term Structure	Definition
postictal	pōst-ik'təl	post = after ictal = relating to or caused by a stroke or seizure	Following a seizure
psychotherapy	si"ko-ther'ə-pe	psych/o = mind or soul therapy = treatment	Treatment of emotional, behavioral, personality, and psychiatric disorders
quadriplegia	kwod"rĭ-ple'jə	quadr/i = four plegia = paralysis	Paralysis of all four limbs
schizophrenia	skiz" o-fre'ne-ə	schiz/o = split phren/o = mind or diaphragm ia = condition of	A type of psychosis in which the mind is said to be split from reality
somatopsychic	so"mə-to-si'kik	somat/o = body psych = mind or soul ic = pertaining to	Relating to the body-mind relationship; the study of the effects of the body upon the mind

Common Medical Terms and Definitions by Body System

Cardiovascular System

Term	Phonetic Spelling	Term Structure	Definition
angiography	an"je-og'rə-fe	angi/o = vessel graphy = process of recording	An examination of blood vessels via radiographic study
anoxia	ə-nok'se-ə	an = not; without oxi = oxygen	Without oxygen
arteriogram	ahr-tēr'-e-o-gram	arteri/o = artery gram = record	Record (X-ray) of an artery
arteriosclerosis	ahr-tēr"e-o-sklə-ro'sis	arteri/o = artery scler/o = hard osis = abnormal condition	Thickening, loss of elasticity, and hardening of arterial walls
arteriostenosis	ahr-tēr"e-o-stə-no'sis	arteri/o = artery stenosis = narrowing	Narrowing of the caliber of an artery, either temporary, through vasoconstriction, or permanent, through arteriosclerosis
atherosclerosis	ath"ər-o-sklə-ro'-sis	ather/o = fat; fatty plaque sclerosis = hardening	The buildup of fatty substances that harden within the walls of arteries
bradycardia	brad"e-kahr'de-ə	brady = slow cardi/o = heart ia = pertaining to	Pertaining to a slow heart rate
cardiologist	kahr"de-ol'ə-jist	cardi/o = heart logist = specialist in the study or treatment of	A physician who specializes in diseases of the heart
cardiomegaly	kahr"de-o-meg'ə-le	cardi/o = heart megaly = enlargement	Enlarged heart
cardiomyopathy	kahr"de-o-mi-op'ə-the	cardi/o = heart my/o = muscle pathy = disease	Disease of the heart muscle
cardiorrhexis	kahr"de-o-rek'sis	cardi/o = heart rhexis = rupture	Rupture of the heart wall

(continued)

Term	Phonetic Spelling	Term Structure	Definition
coronaritis	kor'ə-nar"ī-tis	coron/o = heart itis = inflammation	Inflammation of coronary artery or arteries
diplocardia	dip"lo-kahr'de-ə	diplo = two; double cardi/o = heart ia = pertaining to	Pertaining to an anomaly in which the left and right halves of the heart are separated to varying degrees by a central fissure
endarterectomy	end-ahr"tər-ek'tə-me	end/o = within; in arter/o = artery ectomy = surgical removal; excision	Surgical removal of the inside of an artery
endocardium	en"do-kahr'de-um	endo = within; in cardi/o = heart ium = structure; tissue	Membrane lining the cavities of the heart
hypertension	hi"pər-ten'shən	hyper = above or excessive tension	High blood pressure
hypoxemia	hi"pok-se'me-ə	hypo = below or deficient ox/e = oxygen emia = blood	Too little oxygen in the blood
infracardiac	in"frə-kahr'de-ak	infra = below; inferior cardi/o = heart iac = pertaining to	Beneath the heart; below the level of the heart
myocarditis	mi"o-kahr-di'tis	my/o = muscle cardi/o = heart itis = inflammation	Inflammation of the heart muscle
myocardium	mi"o-kahr'de-əm	my/o = muscle cardi/o = heart ium = structure; tissue	Heart muscle tissue
pericardium	per"ī-kahr'de-əm	peri = around; surrounding cardi/o = heart ium = structure; tissue	Lining around the outside of the heart
sphygmocardiograph	sfig"-mo-kahr'de-o-graf	sphygm/o = pulse cardi/o =heart graph = instrument for recording	A polygraph recording both the heartbeat and the radial pulse
tachycardia	tak"ī-kahr'de-ə	tachy = fast cardi/o = heart ia = pertaining to	Pertaining to a fast heart rate
tricuspid	tri-kus'pid	tri = three cuspid = having one cusp (a leaflet of one of the heart's valves)	Having three points, prongs, or cusps, as the tricuspid valve of the heart

Respiratory System

Term	Phonetic Spelling	Term Structure	Definition
bronchitis	brong-ki'tis	bronch/o = bronchus itis = inflammation	Inflammation of the bronchi
bronchiolitis	brong"ke-o-li'tis	bronchiol/o = bronchiole itis = inflammation	Inflammation of the bronchioles

Respiratory System (continued)

Term	Phonetic Spelling	Term Structure	Definition
bronchoscopy	brong-kos'kə-pe	bronch/o = bronchus scopy = process of viewing	Process of viewing the bronchi
dyspnea	disp'ne-ə	dys = difficult; painful pnea = breathing	Difficult, painful, or faulty breathing
hypoxia	hi-pok'se-ə	hypo = deficient or below oxi = oxygen ia = condition of	A condition of deficient oxygen levels
isocapnia	i"so-kap'-ne'ə	iso = same; equal capnia = carbon dioxide	A state in which the arterial carbon dioxide pressure remains constant or unchanged
laryngoscope	lə-ring'gə-skōp	laryng/o = larynx scope = instrument for viewing	Instrument for viewing the larynx
laryngospasm	lə-ring'go-spaz"əm	laryng/o = larynx spasm = involuntary contraction or twitch	Contraction of laryngeal muscles, causing constriction
pharyngitis	far"in-ji'tis	pharyng/o = pharynx itis = inflammation	Inflammation of the pharynx
pneumothorax	noo"mo-thor'aks	pneum/o = air or lungs thorax = chest; pleural cavity	Air or gas in the chest cavity
pulmonologist	pool"mə-nol'ə-jist	pulmon/o = lungs logist = specialist in the study or treatment of	Specialist in diseases of the lungs
rhinoplasty	ri'no-plas"te	rhin/o = nose plasty = surgical repair	Surgical repair of the nose
rhinorrhea	ri"no-re'ə	rhin/o = nose rrhea = flow; discharge	Discharge from the nose
sinusitis	si"nə-si'tis	sinus/o = sinus itis = inflammation	Inflammation of the mucous membrane of any sinus, especially of one of the paranasal sinuses
spirometry	spi-rom'ə-tre	spir/o = breathe; breath metry = process of measuring	Measurement of breathing
stethoscope	steth'o-skōp	steth/o = chest scope = instrument for viewing	Instrument used to listen to lung and heart sounds through the chest wall
thoracotomy	thor"ə-kot'ə-me	thorac/o = chest otomy = incision into	Incision into the chest
tracheostomy	tra"ke-os'tə-me	trache/o = trachea stomy = creation of an opening	Creation of an opening in the trachea, usually to insert a tube

Musculoskeletal System

Term	Phonetic Spelling	Term Structure	Definition
arthralgia	ahr-thral'jə	arthr/o = joint algia = pain	Joint pain
arthritis	ahr-thri'tis	arthr/o = joint itis = inflammation	Inflammation of the joints

(continued)

Term	Phonetic Spelling	Term Structure	Definition
arthrodesis	ahr"thro-de'sis	arthr/o = joint desis = binding together	The binding together or stiffening of a joint by operative means
arthroscopy	ahr-thros'kə-pe	arthr/o = joint scopy = process of viewing	Process of viewing a joint
bradykinesia	brad"e-kĭ-ne'zhə	brady = slow kinesi/o= movement	Slow movement
bursitis	bər-si'tis	burs/o = joint itis = inflammation	Inflammation of the bursa, a fluid-filled sac around joints
carpopedal	kahr"po-ped'əl	carp/o = wrist bones pedal = relating to the feet	Relating to the wrist and the foot, or the hands and feet
chondromalacia	kon"dro-mə-la'shə	chondro = cartilage malacia = softening	Softening of the cartilage
craniotomy	kra"ne-ot'ə-me	crani/o = cranium; skull otomy = incision into	Surgical incision of the skull
electromyogram	e-lek"tro-mi'o-gram	electr/o = electricity my/o = muscle gram = record	Record of the electrical activity of a muscle
fibulocalcaneal	fib"u-lo-kal-ka'-ne-əl	fibul/o = fibula calcaneus = the largest of the tarsal bones	Relating to the fibula and the calcaneus
hypertrophy	hi-pər'tro-fe	hyper = above; excessive trophy = grown; development	Increase in the size of tissue, such as muscle
intercostal	in"tər-kos'təl	inter = between cost/o = rib al = pertaining to	Pertaining to between the ribs
intramuscular	in"trə-mus'ku-lər	intra = within muscul/o = muscle ar = pertaining to	Pertaining to within the muscle
ligamentopexy	lig"ə-men"to-pek'se	ligament/o = ligament pexy = suspension or fixation	Shortening of any ligament of the uterus
lumbosacral	lum"bo-sa'krəl	lumb/o = lower back sacrum = the segment of the vertebral column forming part of the pelvis	Relating to the lumbar vertebrae and the sacrum
metacarpectomy	met"ə-kahr-pek'tə-me	metacarp/o = hand bones ectomy = surgical removal; excision	Excision of one or all of the metacarpals
metatarsalgia	met"ə-tahr-sal'je	metatars/o = foot bones algia = pain	Pain in the forefoot in the region of the heads of the metatarsals
myalgia	mi-al'jə	my/o = muscle algia = pain	Muscle pain
orthopedic	or"tho-pe'dik	orth/o = straight podi = foot ic = pertaining to	Literally means pertaining to straight foot (ie, pertaining to the study of diseases of the skeletal and muscular system)
orthopedist	or"tho-pe'dist	orth/o = straight podi = foot logist = specialist in the study or treatment of	A specialist in the study of diseases of the skeletal and muscular system

Musculoskeletal System

Term	Phonetic Spelling	Term Structure	Definition
osteomyelitis	os″te-o-mi″ə-li′tis	oste/o = bone myel/o = bone marrow or spinal cord itis = inflammation	Inflammation of the bone and bone marrow
patellectomy	pat″ə-lek′tə-me	patell/o = kneecap ectomy = surgical removal; excision	Surgical removal of the kneecap
pectoralgia	pek′-tə-ral′je	pector/o = chest algia = pain	Pain in the chest
pelviscope	pel′vĭ-skōp	pelv/i = pelvis scope = instrument for viewing	Endoscopic instrument for examining the interior of the pelvis
retroflexion	ret″ro-flek′shən	retro = behind; backward; upward flexion = the act of flexing or bending	Backward bending
rheumatologist	roo″mə-tol′ə-jist	rheum = watery discharge logist = specialist in the study or treatment of	A specialist in rheumatology
spondylolysis	spon″də-lol′ĭ-sis	spondyl/o = vertebra; vertebral column lysis = break down	Degeneration or deficient development of a portion of the vertebra
suprapubic	soo″prə-pu′bik	supra = above; on top of pub/o = pubic bone; pubis ic = pertaining to	Pertaining to above the pubic bone
synovitis	sin″o-vi′tis	synovi/o = joint itis = inflammation	Inflammation of a synovial membrane, especially that of a joint
tarsometatarsal	tahr′so-met″ə-tahr′səl	tars/o = ankle bones metatarsal = any one of the metatarsal bones	Relating to the tarsal and metatarsal bones; denoting the articulations between the two sets of bones
tendinitis	ten″dĭ-ni′tis	tendin/o = tendon itis = inflammation	Inflammation of the tendon

Endocrine System

Term	Phonetic Spelling	Term Structure	Definition
adenoma	ad″ə-no′mə	aden/o = gland oma = tumor	Tumor of glandular tissue
adrenomegaly	ə-dre″no-meg′ə-le	adren/o = adrenal gland megaly = enlargement	Enlargement of the adrenal gland
andromorphous	an″dro-mor′fəs	andr/o = male morph/o = form; shape ous = pertaining to	Male form or appearance
endocrinology	en″do-krĭ-nol′ə-je	end/o = within; in crine = to secrete logy = study of	Study of the secreting glands that comprise the endocrine system

(continued)

Term	Phonetic Spelling	Term Structure	Definition
gonadotropin	go′nə-do-tro″pin	gonad/o = sex glands tropin = nourish; develop; stimulate	A hormone capable of promoting gonadal growth and function
glucogenic	gloo″ko-jen′ik	gluc/o = glucose; sugar genic = origin; producing; forming	Giving rise to or producing glucose
hormonal	hor-mo′nəl	hormone/o = hormone; an urging on al = pertaining to	Pertaining to hormones
hyperglycemia	hi″pər-gli-se′me-ə	hyper = above or excessive glyc/o = glucose; sugar emia = blood	Too much sugar in the blood
hyperthyroidism	hi″pər-thi′roid-iz-əm	hyper = above or excessive thyr/o = thyroid gland ism = condition	Condition of too much thyroid hormone
hypokalemia	hi″po-kə-le′me-ə	hypo = below or deficient kal/i = potassium emia = blood	Low blood potassium
hyposecretion	hi″po-sə-kre′shən	hypo = below or deficient secretion	Abnormally decreased secretion
ketoacidosis	ke″to-as″ĭ-do′sis	ket/o = ketone bodies acid osis = abnormal condition	Condition of an increased presence of ketone bodies
microcytosis	mi″kro-si-to′sis	Micro = small cyt/o = cell osis = abnormal condition	Presence of large red blood cells
pancreatitis	pan″kre-ə-ti′tis	pancreat/o = pancreas itis = inflammation	Inflammation of the pancreas
polydipsia	pol″ĭ-dip′se-ə	poly = many or excessive dips/o = thirst ia = condition of	Condition of excessive thirst
thymoma	thi-mo′mə	thym/o = thymus gland oma = tumor	Tumor of thymic tissue
thyroidectomy	thi″roi-dek′tə-me	thyr/o = thyroid gland ectomy = surgical removal; excision	Surgical removal of the thyroid gland

Immune System

Term	Phonetic Spelling	Term Structure	Definition
anti-inflammatory	an″te-in-flam′ə-to″re	anti = against inflammatory = pertaining to, characterized by, causing, resulting from, or becoming affected by inflammation	Reducing inflammation by acting on body responses, without directly antagonizing the causative agent
autoimmune	aw″to-ĭ-mūn′	auto = self immune/o = protection	The disorder characterized by abnormal function of the immune system that causes the body to produce antibodies against itself

Immune System (continued)

Term	Phonetic Spelling	Term Structure	Definition
calcipenia	kal"sī-pe'ne-ə	calc/i = calcium penia = decreased number	A condition in which there is an insufficient amount of calcium in the tissues and fluids of the body
carcinogenic	kahr"sin-o-jen'ik	carcin/o = cancerous genic = origin; producing; forming	Causing cancer
immunocompromised	im"u-no-kom'prə-mīzd	immune/o = protection compromised	A condition in which the immune system has been compromised by disease or immunosuppressive agents
leukemia	loo-ke'me-ə	leuk/o = white emia = blood	A malignant blood disease marked by abnormal white blood cells or leukocytes
lymphadenopathy	lim-fad"ə-nop'ə-the	lymph/o = lymph aden/o = gland pathy = disease	A disease state in which lymph nodes are enlarged
lymphocytopenia	lim"fo-si"to-pe'ne-ə	lymph/o = lymph cyt/o = cell penia = decreased number	An abnormally reduced number of lymphocytes
lymphoma	lim-fo'mə	lymph/o = lymph oma = tumor	A neoplasm of the lymphatic system
macrocytosis	mak"ro-si-to'sis	macro = large cytosis = condition of cells	The presence of large red blood cells
metastasis	mə-tas'tə-sis	meta = beyond; after; change stasis = stop or control	The spread of cancer cells beyond the original site of the tumor through blood or lymph
pancytopenia	pan"si-to-pe'ne-ə	pan = all cyt/o = cell penia = decreased number	An abnormally reduced number of all types of blood cells
phagocyte	fag'o-sīt	phag/o = eat or swallow cyt/o = cell	A cell that consumes bacteria, foreign particles, and other cells
rhabdomyoma	rab"do-mi-o'mə	rhabdomy/o = skeletal muscle; striated muscle oma = tumor	A benign neoplasm derived from striated muscle
septicemia	sep"tĭ-se'me-ə	septi =bacteria emia = blood	Bacterial infection of the blood
splenomegaly	sple"no-meg'ə-le	splen/o = spleen megaly = enlargement	An enlarged spleen
thymus	thi'məs	thym/o = thymus gland ectomy = surgical removal; excision	The removal of the thymus gland

Hematologic System

Term	Phonetic Spelling	Term Structure	Definition
adipocyte	ad'ĭ-po-sīt"	adip/o = fat cyte = cell	Fat cell

(continued)

Term	Phonetic Spelling	Term Structure	Definition
anemia	ə-ne′me-ə	an = not; without emia = blood	A blood condition in which there is a reduction in the number of red blood cells, hemoglobin, or the volume of packed red blood cells
arteriolonecrosis	ahr-tēr″e-o″lo-nə-kro′sis	arteriol/o = arteriole necrosis = pathologic death of one or more cells or of a portion of tissue or organ	Death of arterioles
coagulopathy	ko-ag″u-lop′ə-the	coagul/o = clotting pathy = disease	A disease affecting the coagulability of the blood
eosinopenia	e″o-sin-o-pe′ne-ə	eosin/o = red penia = decreased number	The presence of eosinophils in an abnormally small number in the peripheral bloodstream
erythrocyte	ə-rith′ro-sīt	erythro = red cyte = cell	A mature red blood cell
glomerulopathy	glo-mer″u-lop′ə-the	glomerul/o = glomerulus pathy = disease	Glomerular disease of any type
hemangioma	he-man″je-o′mə	hemangi/o = blood vessel oma = tumor	A congenital anomaly in which proliferation of blood vessels leads to a mass that resembles a neoplasm
hematocrit	he-mat′ə-krit	hemat/o = blood crit = to separate	Percentage of the volume of a blood sample occupied by cells
hematology	he″mə-tol′ə-je	hemat/o = blood logy = study of	Medical study of the blood
hemocytoblasts	he″mo-si′to-blasts	hem/o = blood cyt/o = cell blast = germ or bud	Primitive cells in the bone marrow that develop into blood cells
hemoglobin	he′mo-glo″bin	hem/o = blood globin = protein	The protein-iron compound in erythrocytes that transports oxygen and carbon dioxide
hemolysis	he-mol′ə-sis	hem/o = blood lysis = break down	The breakdown of the red blood cell membrane
hematopoiesis	he″mə-to-, hem″ə-to-poi-e′sis	hem/o = blood poiesis = formation	The process of formation and development of various types of blood cells
ileopexy	il″e-o-peck-se	ile/o = ileum pexy = suspension or fixation	Surgical fixation of the ileum
leukopenia	loo″ko-pe′ne-ə	leuko = white penia = decreased number	Too few white blood cells
lipoid	lip′oid	lip/o = fat oid = resembling; like	Resembling fat
morphology	mor-fol′ə-je	morph/o = form; shape logy = study of	The study of form, including the size and shape of a specimen, such as a blood cell
myeloma	mi″ə-lo′mə	myel/o = bone marrow or spinal cord oma = tumor	Tumor of the bone marrow
myelocyte	mi′ə-lo-sīt	myel/o = bone marrow or spinal cord cyt/o = cell	An immature blood cell in the bone marrow

Hematologic System (continued)

Term	Phonetic Spelling	Term Structure	Definition
reticulocyte	rə-tik'u-lo-sīt"	reticul/o = a net cyt/o = cell	Immature red blood cells or erythrocytes
spherocyte	sfēr'o-sit	sphere/o = round cyte = cell	A small, spherical red blood cell
thrombophlebitis	throm"bo-flə-bi'tis	thromb/o = clot phleb/o = vein itis = inflammation	Inflammation of a vein due to blood clot formation

Gastrointestinal System

Term	Phonetic Spelling	Term Structure	Definition
abdominocentesis	ab-dom"ĭ-no-sen-te'sis	abdomin/o = abdomen centesis = surgical puncture	A puncture of the abdomen for aspiration of abdominal fluid
biligenesis	bil"ĭ-jen'ə-sis	bili = bile genesis = origin; producing; forming	Bile production
buccolingual	buk"o-ling'gwəl	bucc/o = cheek lingual = tongue	Pertaining to the cheek and tongue
cholangiogram	ko-lan'je-o-gram	cholangi/o = bile duct gram = record	The radiographic record of the bile ducts obtained by cholangiography
cholecystectomy	ko"le-sis-tek'tə-me	cholecyst/o = gall bladder ectomy = surgical removal; excision	Surgical removal of the gall bladder
cirrhosis	sĭ-ro'sis	cirrh/o = yellow osis = abnormal condition	Chronic liver condition that causes yellowing of tissues
colonoscopy	ko"lon-os'kə-pe	col/o = colon scopy = process of viewing	Process of viewing the colon
dentalgia	den-tal'jə	dent = tooth algia = pain	Dental pain (toothache)
duodenotomy	doo"o-də-not'ə-me	duoden/o = duodenum otomy = incision into	Incision of the duodenum
dyspepsia	dis-pep'se-ə	dys = difficult; painful pepsia = digestion	The condition of indigestion or of painful digestion
dysphagia	dis-fa'je-ə	dys = difficult; painful phag/o = eat or swallow ia = pertaining to	Pertaining to difficulty in eating or swallowing
endoscopic	en"do-skop'ik	end/o = within; in scopy = process of viewing ic = pertaining to	Pertaining to the process of viewing within
esophagitis	ə-sof"ə-ji'tis	esophag/o = esophagus itis = inflammation	Inflammation of the esophagus
gastroenterologist	gas"tro-en"tər-ol'ə-jist	gastro = stomach enter/o = intestines ologist = specialist in the study or treatment of	Specialist in the study or treatment of the stomach and intestines
gingivitis	jin"jĭ-vi'tis	gingiv/o = gums itis = inflammation	Inflammation of the gingiva as a response to bacterial plaque on adjacent teeth

(continued)

Term	Phonetic Spelling	Term Structure	Definition
glossology	glos-ol'ə-je	gloss/o = tongue logy = study of	The branch of medical science concerned with the tongue and its diseases
hematemesis	he"mə-tem'ə-sis	hemat/o = blood emesis = vomit	Bloody vomit
hepatomegaly	hep"ə-to-meg'ə-le	hepat/o = liver megaly = enlargement	Enlargement of the liver
jejunoplasty	jə"joo-no-plas"te	jejun/o = jejunum plasty = surgical repair	A corrective surgical procedure on the jejunum
laparomyositis	lap"ə-ro-mi-o'tis	lapar/o = abdominal wall my/o = muscle itis = inflammation	Inflammation of the lateral abdominal muscles
malocclusion	mal"o-kloo'zhən	mal = bad; poor; abnormal occlusion = the act of closing or the state of being closed	Any deviation from a physiologically acceptable contact of opposing dentitions
mucolytic	mu"ko-lit'ik	muc/o = mucus lytic = break down	Capable of dissolving, digesting, or liquefying mucus
nasogastric	na"zo-gas'trik	nas/o = nose gastr/o = stomach ic = pertaining to	Pertaining to the nose and the stomach (eg, a tube that travels from the nose to the stomach)
noncariogenic	non-kahr"sin-o-jen'ik	non = not caries = destruction or necrosis of teeth (cavity) genic = origin; producing; forming	Not caries-producing
pancreatitis	pan"kre-ə-ti'tis	pancreat/o = pancreas itis = inflammation	Inflammation of the pancreas
proctostenosis	prok"to-stə-no'sis	proct/o = rectum stenosis = narrowing	Stricture of the rectum or anus
rectocele	rek'to-sēl	rect/o = rectum cele = hernia; herniation	Pouching of the rectum into the vagina
sialometry	si"ə'-lo-met-re	sial/o = saliva metry = process of measuring	A measurement of salivary secretion
stomatitis	sto"mə-ti'tis	stomat/o = mouth itis = inflammation	Inflammation of the mucous membrane of the mouth
sublingual	səb-ling'gwəl	sub = below; under lingua = tongue al = pertaining to	Pertaining to under the tongue

Urinary System

Term	Phonetic Spelling	Term Structure	Definition
bacteriuria	bak-tēr"e-u're-ə	bacteri/o = bacteria ur/o = urinary tract ia = a condition of	The presence of bacteria in the urine
cystoscope	sis'to-skōp"	cyst/o = sac or bladder scope = instrument for viewing	Type of endoscope that is used to examine the bladder

Urinary System (continued)

Term	Phonetic Spelling	Term Structure	Definition
glucosuria	gloo"ko-su're-ə	gluc/o = glucose; sugar ur/o = urinary tract ia = a condition of	A condition of sugar in the urine
hydronephrosis	hi"dro-nə-fro'sis	hydr/o = water; fluid nephr/o = kidney osis = abnormal condition	A condition of urine pooling in the renal pelvis
ketonuria	ke"to-nu're-ə	ket/o = ketone bodies ur/o = urinary tract ia = condition of	Condition of ketone bodies in the urine
lithotripsy	lith'o-trip"se	lith/o = stone tripsy = crushing	The crushing of a stone
nephrectomy	nə-frek'tə-me	nephr/o = kidney ectomy = surgical removal; excision	Surgical removal of a kidney
nephrosis	nĕ-fro'sis	nephr/o = kidney osis = abnormal condition	An abnormal condition of the kidney
polyuria	pol"e-u're-ə	poly = many or excessive ur/o = urinary tract ia = condition of	Condition in which one urinates excessively
pyelonephritis	pi"ə-lo-nə-fri'tis	pyel/o = renal pelvis nephr/o = kidney itis = inflammation	Inflammation of the renal pelvis area of the kidney
renogenic	re"no-jen'ik	ren/o = kidney genic = origin; producing; forming	Originating in the kidney
ureterolithiasis	u-re"tər-o-lĭ-thi'ə-sis	ureter/o = ureter lith/o = stone iasis = formation of; presence of	The condition of having a stone form in the ureter
urethralgia	u"re-thral'jə	urethr/o = urethra algia = pain	Pain in the urethra
urologist	u-rol'ə-jist	ur/o = urinary tract logist = a specialist in the study or treatment of	Physician who specializes in conditions of the urinary system
vesicotomy	ves"ĭ-kot'ə-me	vesic/o = sac or bladder otomy = incision into	An incision into the bladder

Other Body Systems

Section I: The Eyes

Term	Phonetic Spelling	Term Structure	Definition
blepharitis	blef"ə-ri'tis	blephar/o = eyelid itis = inflammation	Inflammation of the eyelid
conjunctivitis	kən-junk"tĭ-vi'tis	conjunctiv/o = conjunctiva itis = inflammation	Inflammation of the conjunctiva
exophthalmia	ek"sof-thal'me-ə	ex/o = out ophthalm/o = eye ia = pertaining to	Pertaining to a protuberance of the eye

Term	Phonetic Spelling	Term Structure	Definition
glaucoma	glaw-ko′mə	glauc/o = silver; gray oma = tumor	A disease of the eye characterized by increased intraocular pressure, excavation, and atrophy of the optic nerve; produces defects in the field of vision
intraocular	in″trə-ok′u-lər	intra = within ocul/o = eye ar = pertaining to	Pertaining to the inside of the eye
keratoplasty	ker′ə-to-plas″te	kerat/o = cornea plasty = surgical repair	The surgical repair or reconstruction of the cornea
lacrimation	lak″rĭ-ma′shən	lacrim/o = tears ation = a process	The process of secreting tears
ophthalmologist	of″thəl-mol′ə-jist	ophthalm/o = eye ologist = specialist in the study or treatment of	Specialist in diseases of the eye
optometry	op-tom′ə-tre	opt/o = eye metry = process of measuring	Process of measuring the eye
photophobia	fo″to-fo′be-ə	phot/o = light phobia = abnormal fear	Extreme sensitivity and discomfort from light
presbyopia	pres″be-o′pe-ə	presby/o = old age opia = a condition of vision	A vision condition of a reduced ability to focus due to old age
retinitis	ret″ĭ-ni′tis	retin/o = retina itis = inflammation	Inflammation of the retina

Section II: The Ears

Term	Phonetic Spelling	Term Structure	Definition
audiometry	aw″de-om′ə-tre	audi/o = hearing; sound metry = measurement	Measurement of hearing
auriculocranial	aw-rik″u-lo-kra′-ne-əl	aur/o = ear cranium = the bones of the head	Relating to the auricle or pinna of the ear and the cranium
cochleitis	kok″le-i′tis	cochle/o = cochlea itis = inflammation	Inflammation of the cochlea
myringitis	mir″in-ji′tis	myring/o = eardrum itis = inflammation	Inflammation of the tympanic membrane
otorhinolaryngologist	o″to-ri″no-lar″in-gol′ə-jist	ot/o = ear rhin/o = nose laryng/o = larynx ologist = specialist in the study or treatment of	Specialist in diseases of the ear, nose, and throat
otalgia	o-tal′je-ə	ot/o = ear algia = pain	Earache
otitis	o-ti′tis	ot/o = ear itis = inflammation	Inflammation of the ear
otosclerosis	o″to-sklə-ro′sis	ot/o = ear sclerosis = hardening	A condition of hardening of bone tissue in the ear

Section II: The Ears (continued)

Term	Phonetic Spelling	Term Structure	Definition
presbyacusis	pres"be-ə-ku'-sis	presby/o = old age acous/o = a hearing condition	Hearing loss due to old age
salpingitis	sal"pin-ji'tis	salping/o = eustachian or uterine tube itis = inflammation	Inflammation of the eustachian tube in the ear or the uterine tube
tympanometry	tim"pə-nom'ə-tre	tympan/o = eardrum metry = the process of measuring	The process of measuring the compliance and mobility (conductibility) of the tympanic membrane
tympanoplasty	tim"pə-no-plas'te	tympan/o = eardrum plasty = surgical repair	Surgical repair of the eardrum

Section III: The Dermatologic System

Term	Phonetic Spelling	Term Structure	Definition
dermatitis	der"mə-ti'tis	dermat/o = skin itis = inflammation	Inflammation of the skin
dermatologist	dər"mə-tol'o-jĭst	dermat/o = skin ologist = specialist in the study or treatment of	Specialist in the study of diseases of the skin
epidermal	ep"ĭ-dər'məl	epi = on; upon derm/o = skin al = pertaining to	Pertaining to on the skin
histology	his-tol'ə-je	hist/o = tissue logy = study of	The study of tissues
keratosis	ker"ə-to'sis	kerat/o = hard osis = abnormal condition	A condition of thickened epidermis
melanoderma	mel'ə-no-der'mə	melan/o = black derma = skin	An abnormal darkening of the skin by deposition of excess melanin
onychomycosis	on"ĭ-ko-mi-ko'sis	onych/o = nail myc/o = fungus osis = abnormal condition	Fungal infection of the nail
pachyderma	pak"e-der'mə	pachy = thick derma = skin	Abnormally thick skin
percutaneous	per"ku-ta'ne-əs	per = through cutane/o = skin ous = pertaining to	Through the skin
sarcoma	sahr"ko'mə	sarc/o = flesh oma = tumor	Tumor of the flesh
subcutaneous	sub"ku-ta'ne-əs	sub = below; under cutane/o = skin ous = pertaining to	Pertaining to below the skin
xanthoderma	zan"tho-der'mə	xanth/o = yellow derma = skin	Any yellow coloration of the skin
xeroderma	zēr"o-der'mə	xero = dry derm/o = skin	Dry skin

Section IV: Reproductive System

Term	Phonetic Spelling	Term Structure	Definition
amniocentesis	am″ne-o-sen-te′-sis	amni/o = amnion centesis = surgical puncture	Aspiration of a small amount of amniotic fluid for analysis of possible fetal abnormalities
anorchism	an-or′kiz-əm	an = not; without orch/o = testis; testicle ism = condition	The condition in which one or both testes are absent
antenatal	an″te-na′təl	ante = before; forward natal = relating to birth	The time before birth, also known as the prenatal period
aspermia	ə-spər′me-ə	a = not; without sperm/o = sperm ia = condition of	The condition in which one is unable to produce or ejaculate sperm
contraception	kon″trə-sep-shən	contra = against; opposite conception = act of conceiving; the implantation of the blastocyte in the endometrium	Prevention of conception or impregnation
colposcope	kol′po-skōp	colp/o = vagina (sheath) scope = instrument for viewing	A special kind of scope designed to examine the vagina
ectopic	ek-top′ik	ect = outside; out top/o = place ic = pertaining to	Out of place; said of an organ not in its proper position, or of a pregnancy occurring elsewhere than in the cavity of the uterus
embryoblast	em′bre-o-blast″	embry/o = embryo blast = germ or bud	The cells at the embryonic pole of the blastocyst concerned with formation of the body of the embryo
epididymitis	ep″ĭ-did′ə-mi′tis	epididym/o = epididymis itis = inflammation	Inflammation of the epididymis
episiotomy	ə-piz″e-ot′o-me	episi/o = vulva tomy = incision into	An incision made in the perineum to facilitate childbirth
gynecologist	gi″nə-kol′ə-jist″	gynec/o = woman logist = a specialist in the study or treatment of	A physician who specializes in the reproductive system of women
hydrocele	hi′dro-sēl	hydr/o = water or fluid cele = hernia or herniation	A hernia of fluid in the testis or tubes leading from the testis
hysterectomy	his″tər-ek′tə-me	hyster/o = uterus ectomy = surgical removal; excision	The surgical removal of the uterus
lactogenic	lak″to-jen′ik	lact/o = milk genic = origin; producing; forming	Pertaining to the production of milk
mammogram	mam′ə-gram	mamm/o = breast gram = record	An X-ray of the breast
mastodynia	mas″to-din′e-ə	mast/o = breast dynia = pain	Breast pain
menorrhalgia	men″o-ral′jə	men/o = menses; menstruation r/rhage = bursting forth algia = pain	Difficult and painful menstruation

Section IV: Reproductive System (continued)

Term	Phonetic Spelling	Term Structure	Definition
neonatal	ne″o-na′təl	neo = new nat/o = birth; delivery al = pertaining to	Pertaining to newborn
obstetrics	ob-stet′riks	obstetr/o = midwife ic = pertaining to	The specialty pertaining to the care and treatment of mother and fetus throughout pregnancy, childbirth, and the immediate postpartum period
oligospermia	ol″ĭ-go-sper′me-ə	oligo = few or less sperm/o = sperm	Too few sperm in the semen
oophoritis	o″of-ə-ri′tis	oophor/o = ovary itis = inflammation	Inflammation of the ovary
orchiopexy	or″ke-o-pek′se	orchi/o = testis; testicle pexy = suspension or fixation	Surgical treatment of an undescended testicle by freeing it and implanting it into the scrotum
prostatalgia	pros″tə-tal′jə	prostat/o = prostate algia = pain	Painful prostate
vasectomy	və-sek′tə-me	vas/o = vessel ectomy = surgical removal; excision	Excision of part of the vas deferens to produce male sterility

Appendix B

Common Formulations and Conversions

Common Roman Numerals:

ss = ½ I or i = 1 V or v = 5 X or x = 10
L or l = 50 C or c = 100 M or m = 1000

Metric System Conversions

WEIGHTS

1 kilogram (kg) = 1000 gm
1 gram (gm or g) = 1000 mg
1 milligram (mg) = 1000 mcg

VOLUME

1 Liter (L) = 1000 mL
1 milliliter (mL) = 1000 microliters

DISTANCE

1 Kilometer (km) = 1000 meters (m)
1 m = 100 centimeters (cm) = 1000 millimeters (mm)

Converting Measures of Length

Metric	Household System
2.54 cm	1 inch

Converting Measures of Mass / Weight

Metric	Avoirdupois / Apothecary
1 kilogram (kg)	2.2 pounds (lb)
454 g	1 lb
28.4 g (usually rounded to 30 g)	1 ounce
60 mg	1 grain (Apothecary system)

Converting Measures of Volume

Metric	Household System
5 mL	1 teaspoon (tsp)
15 mL	1 tablespoon (T)
30 mL	1 fluid ounce (fl oz)
473 mL (usually rounded to 480 mL)	1 pint
3785 mL or 3.785L (usually rounded to 3800 mL or 3.8L)	1 gallon

Converting Within the Household System

1 cup	8 fluid ounces
2 cups	1 pint = 16 fluid ounces
2 pints	1 quart = 32 fluid ounces
4 quarts	1 gallon = 128 fluid ounces

Converting Temperature

To convert Fahrenheit temperature (T_F) to Celsius temperature (T_C):

$$T_C = \frac{5}{9} \times (T_F - 32)$$

To convert Celsius temperature (T_C) to Fahrenheit temperature (T_F):

$$T_F = \frac{9}{5} \times (T_C + 32)$$

Body Surface Area (BSA)

The Mosteller formula:

$$BSA\,(m^2) = \sqrt{\frac{[height(cm) \times weight\,(kg)]}{3600}}$$

Ideal Body Weight (IBW)

IBW (kg) for males = 50 kg + 2.3 (inches over 5')
IBW (kg) for females = 45.5 kg + 2.3 (inches over 5')

Body Mass Index (BMI)

$$BMI\left(\frac{kg}{m^2}\right) = \frac{weight\,(kg)}{[height\,(m)]^2}$$

Index